You're Not Aging...
You're Just Oxidizing!

You're Not Aging, You're Just Oxidizing

By Tom Porter
Copyright 2004

Malibu Wellness, Inc.
www.WellnessSalon.com
800.622.7332

EC Mode® products and Malibu 2000 products are
brands of Malibu Wellness, Inc.

Contributors

Carrie Phelps . . . . Editor
June Hagman . . . . Contributing Editor & Testimonials
Deb Porter . . . . Contributing Editor & Researcher
Vitaliy Leonov . . . . Layout & Graphics
RJ Howard . . . . Proofreader
Bill Knapp . . . . Photographer
Lauri Fraser . . . . Stylist

*Dedicated to Deb, my wife and partner,
for her inspiration and motivation; along with
Trevor, our son, who "raises the bar" for
focus, discipline and integrity.*

Table of Contents

Foreword v

Chapter 1 - Introduction 1
Oxidation is all Around You 2
Total Oxidation Management 3
A Life Changing Event Opens a New Door 5
The Evolution of Malibu Wellness 5
Knowledge is Power 6

Chapter 2 - Aging Assumptions 7
Harman's Theory of Aging 7
Genetics & Environment 8
Learning a New Vocabulary 12
Managing Oxidation is Simple 13
Are You Making Assumptions that Might Cause You
to Appear to Age Faster? 14
Answering Your Assumptions 15

Chapter 3 - The Root of Oxidation 19
Putting the Brakes on Aging 19
Oxygen: Our "Dangerous Friend" 20
Oxidation with Air, Sun & Water 21
Bleach is Oxidation 22
Play & Exercise—Oxidize! 22
How Your Home & Work Can be Oxidizing Environments 23
How Fast is Your Skin Oxidizing 24

Chapter 4 - The "Cost" of Free Radicals 27
A Closer Look at Free Radicals 28

Chapter 5 - Vitamin C & Vitamin E are Superior 33
Start Fighting the Signs of Aging Today 33
Vitamins: Vita=Vital—It's Life! 34
Cells Absorb Vitamins: Water vs. Oil 35
Understanding the Word Antioxidant 37
Vitamin C is a Superior Antioxidant 39
Vitamin E: an Antioxidant Partner to Vitamin C 45
Vitamin E & Vitamin C are Better Together 50
Other Free Radical Scavengers 51

Chapter 6 - Living "In the Mode" 57

What is "Normal" Skin? 57

"Abnormal" Skin 58

Caring for Your Skin 59

Step 1: 12% L-Ascorbic Acid Form of Vitamin C 60

Step 2: 5% Natural Vitamin E 62

Cleansers, Astringents & Scrubs 63

Chapter 7 - The Air Quality in Your Environment Ages You 69

Oxygen + Environment = Oxidation! 69

Chapter 8 - The Water in Your Environment Ages You 75

Chlorine is All Around You 76

What is Hard Water? 77

You Could Have Hard Water If: 78

Hard Water & Skin 80

The pH of Your Water 80

Measuring pH 82

Chapter 9 - The Sun in Your Environment Ages You 87

Sun is Energy! 88

Suntan vs. Sunburn 90

Tanning Beds, Lamps & Salons 91

Medications Can Create Photo-Toxic &
Photo-Sensitive Allergic Reactions 92

Protecting Your Skin from Sun Damage 93

Chapter 10 - All Sunscreens are Not Created Equal 95

The FDA Creates Stricter Sunscreen Regulations 97

Water & Sweat Resistance Claims on Sunscreens 100

Sunless Tanning Products 101

Adding Vitamins E & C to Sun Protection 101

Chapter 11 - Skin is Simple to Understand 103

The Components of Skin 104

Water Cells 105

Protein Cells: The Physical Building Blocks of Skin 106

Oil/Fat/Lipid Cells: Protecting the Skin's Surface Layers 108

Melanin—The Color of Your "Genes" 108

Dermis & Epidermis: What Lies Beneath 109

The Space Between 110

Epidermis: The Defense Department for the Dermis 111

The Life & Death Cycle of the Epidermis 112

Basal Section 114

Stratum Spinosum: Live Proteins Begin to Die 116

Stratum Granulosum: Dying Cells Begin to Flatten 117

Stratum Lucidum: Hands, Feet, Elbows & Heels 119

Stratum Corneum: A Wall of Dead Brick-like Proteins 120

Chapter 12 - Exfoliation 123

The Second Most Abused Word in Skin Care 123

Normalizing Exfoliation vs. Radical Exfoliation 124

Don't Fool Mother Nature 125

Radical Exfoliation (Resurfacing) is NOT a Lifestyle 126

Normalizing Exfoliation is Total Oxidation Management 127

Chapter 13 - Your Skin Care Professional 129

Plastic Surgeon 130

Dermatologist 130

Esthetician 131

Medical Procedures vs. Cosmetic Beautification 133

Choosing the Right Professional for You 134

Total Oxidation Management: A Bridge Between Doctors & Salons 136

Chapter 14 - Exfoliating Skin Services & Other Treatments ... 139

Radical Exfoliation 139

Because of the damage to the skin, chemical peels
have serious consequences, including: 140

Chemical Peels & How They Work 141

AHA & BHA Chemical Peels 143

AHA's: A List From the FDA 144

Laser Resurfacing or Laser Peels (Light Energy) 153

Exciting New Non–Ablative Light Laser Therapies 155

Dermabrasion: Sanding Away Your Skin 156

Muscle Stimulation 158

Infrared-Light Therapy 158

Oxygen Therapy 159

If You Are Still Planning Radical Exfoliation 160

Post Chemical Peel Care 161

Table of contents

Stages of Healing 162

Summary of Resurfacing: Skin Deep Damage 163

Conclusion **167**

You Are Responsible for Your Skin 167

You're Not Aging...You're Just Oxidizing! 168

Living "In the Mode" 169

Changes You Can Make Now, No Matter How Old You Are 170

Skin Conditions & Testimonials **171**

Acne 173

Age Spots, Keratosis & Comedones 182

Broken Capillaries 186

Burns 189

Chemically Peeled Skin 193

Cradle Cap 198

Contact Dermatitis 201

Dandruff – Itchy, Flaky Scalp 205

Diaper Rash 208

Eczema of the Skin 211

Dry Skin & Irritated Hands 216

Poison Ivy 222

Psoriasis 226

Reconstructive Surgery (Before & After) 232

Rosacea 235

Skin Cancer & Skin Growths 239

Sunburn 244

Swimmers' Oxidation 248

Wounds 251

Wrinkles, Fine Lines & Signs of Aging 255

In Closing **261**

Acknowledgments **a-1**

References **a-3**

Index **a-13**

FOREWORD

Live your life the way you want to remember it,
Live your life the way you want it to be.
Live your life the way you want to remember it,
Live your life inspiring memories.

Don't grow old to regret
The things that you haven't done yet,
Realize...after all of your 'tries,'
If you go for it, that's what you'll get!

Raised in a town outside of Nashville, I believed that a boy from Tennessee was expected to write songs. This excerpt is from a "song" I wrote after college that has remained my mantra—the philosophy of how I live my life.

"If you go for it, that's what you'll get" is an extension of my belief in the concept of "cause and effect." Every action results in a consequence, whether good or bad. Behavior, science, and everything around us have a cause and an effect. This means that you determine your own future by the choices you make.

This book is about making small shifts in behavior—which took me years to discover—that will make big differences in your life. The first twenty-five years of my life, I grew up in an oxidizing world without knowing the long-term consequences. I spent as much time as possible playing outside—including waterskiing, being a lifeguard at pools and at the beach—not knowing what my tanned, and sometimes burned skin, would lead to later in life.

The second twenty-five years of my life, I began asking questions that led to more formal research. Wellness became more important to me. I began pondering questions about how our bodies interact with our environment, and discovered how the correct vitamins in a superior formulation could provide wellness solutions and prevent many serious conditions of the skin, including many signs of aging.

The third twenty-five years of my life has begun with the alarming knowledge of how much damage I did to my skin in the early years. Because I oxidized so much during my first twenty-five years, that early damage is now more visible. The lifestyle I now embrace is a daily wellness approach of reversing those signs of early damage as soon as they appear and prevent future damage from occurring.

I still play outside, I still waterski, but now I am a different kind of lifeguard. Because I am now aware of my responsibility fo the care of my skin, I live a lifestyle of Total Oxidation Management – a lifestyle I am now teaching others.

The fourth twenty-five years of my life will be full of observation. I plan to play more. I plan to live more with the attitude of my first twenty-five years, but with the perspective of my experiences. I am confident that a Total Oxidation Management lifestyle will not only promote how long I live, but also how well I live. It can do the same for you.

Chapter 1

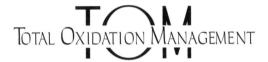

Total Oxidation Management

Introduction

"You're Not Aging, You're Just Oxidizing" will help you understand that you have more control than you may think over how fast your skin shows signs of aging, and also provide you with solutions to common skin conditions that may have been plaguing you for years. You will discover how to make some simple lifestyle shifts that may actually reverse the appearance of wrinkles, fine lines and age spots, as well as help prevent more signs of aging from occurring.

Before you can make those lifestyle changes, however, you first need to understand what "oxidizing" means and how it causes you to age. In later chapters, oxidation will be described in greater detail; for right now, we'll define oxidation as simply the end result of constant and intermittent, aggressive exposure to oxygen—compounded by exposure to elements such as wind, water or sun. A typical example of oxidation is the corrosion or rusting of iron.

Another example of oxidation, and one that is perhaps more applicable to skin, is what I explained to my 19-year-old son when he asked me one day why slowing the aging process is so important. I explained to him that the appearance of our bodies is like a favorite shirt. You probably want that shirt to last and look new as long as it can. Eventually, however, through repeated wearing, washing and drying, that shirt will begin to fade and the fabric will wear out. Think of your skin much like the fabric of that favorite shirt: while outside elements will begin to wear it down, how you care for it depends on how good it looks and how long it lasts.

Oxidation is all Around You

Caring for your skin is challenging, since your body is bombarded every day by common elements in your environment that oxidize your skin. The things you do as you go about your life might actually speed up how fast you appear to age—things as simple as:

- Walking from your office to your car and being exposed to the sun.
- Smoking or being around people who smoke.
- Inhaling exhaust fumes from cars as you walk across the street.
- Taking a shower and being exposed to the chlorine and other chemicals and minerals in the water.

To counteract the results of the environment on our skin, many people turn to popular skin care products and services—yet many of these products and services are either ineffective or can actually be counter-productive. Skin care products, for example, often start out containing the right ingredients to reverse damage and to provide other benefits, but are either ineffectively formulated or left in warehouse boxes so long that those ingredients no longer work by the time the products are purchased. Skin care services, such as chemical peels, are radical approaches that provide short-term fixes with long-term consequences that can actually lead to more severe damage than the original condition.

So, what's the answer to protecting your skin if it is impossible to avoid oxidation, since oxidizers are all around you?

Total Oxidation Management

If oxidation is causing you to age faster, then it just makes sense that you need to manage that oxidation. Free radicals— the culprits that cause aging and which will be explained in further depth later in this book—are caused by oxidation. Free radicals create dysfunctional molecules which lead to unhealthy cells that result in skin appearing old. The purpose of Total Oxidation Management is to prevent the formation of free radicals and to help normalize existing free radicals to prevent them from spreading.

Total Oxidation Management is a lifestyle that incorporates making smart lifestyle choices that minimize overexposure to oxidizing elements along with the daily use of topically applied fresh-dried antioxidant vitamins. As you will read throughout this book, much of Total Oxidation Management centers on the use of the L-ascorbic acid form of Vitamin C and its partner, natural Vitamin E, in ways you may not have considered.

But Total Oxidation Management is not only about products as it is about being mindful of your exposure to oxidation. You will discover how you are uniquely affected by geographical factors, such as what's in your water at home and work, how much sun, snow or rain falls in your area, and by the activities in which you participate.

I became more mindful of oxidation and the aging process while I was pursuing my doctorate in Instructional Systems Technology at Indiana University at Bloomington in the early 1980's. While in Bloomington, I led the development of the

Monroe County YMCA, the largest Wellness Center of its kind in the world.

While we were building this wellness center, I expanded my theories in slowing the aging process by reading research by Linus Pauling on Vitamin C, participating in programs led by Kenneth Cooper at the Cooper Clinic in Dallas, Texas, and by traveling to the Pritikin Longevity Center in Santa Monica, California.

These and other wellness leaders influenced me to open my eyes to nature's methods for defending our bodies to slow the aging process. A member of the wellness center in Bloomington also told me about research on vitamins that was being conducted at Ball State University.

All of this information led to my discovery of research on the benefits of the L-ascorbic acid form of Vitamin C and its fundamental relationship with the body. Some of the most interesting research was led by Ball State University chemist Dr. Keith Ault and the University of Illinois biologist Dr. Joseph Larson, and was the conclusive evidence that Vitamin C plays an important role in the performance and protection of skin cells.

I left the YMCA in Bloomington to move to Malibu, Calif., and still twenty years later, the professionals and community leaders of this unique Wellness Center are serving over 14,000 members with programs that are models for wellness centers worldwide.

It was during the move to Malibu that a life changing event fueled my passion about the benefits of topically applied, freshly-activated antioxidant vitamins. This led me to establish the first company to formulate products containing fresh-dried Vitamin C and Vitamin E for hair and skin care.

A Life Changing Event Opens a New Door

A near fatal car accident in 1982 led me to further explore the benefits of fresh-dried vitamins E and C to accelerate wound healing, slow the signs of aging and manage other common skin conditions. While traveling to Malibu with my wife, Deb, a car accident caused me to crash through the windshield of our car at 60 mph. The emergency room physician who sewed over forty-five stitches into my face told me that I would undoubtedly need the services of a plastic surgeon to perform a series of surgical procedures in the hopes of restoring the original appearance of my face.

I immediately began applying a daily solution of Vitamin C. After the stitches were removed, I began following the Vitamin C with an application of concentrated Vitamin E directly to all affected areas of my face. Two months later at my follow-up visit, the plastic surgeon was surprised at the accelerated healing of my skin. The daily topical application of these active vitamins had accelerated the healing of my skin and had minimized scar tissue, ultimately preventing the need for plastic surgery altogether.

I continued my daily topical vitamin application for the next six years, during which time I was still finding tiny slivers of windshield glass surfacing. Over time, my face began to normalize and the previous signs of damage were no longer visible. Since then, I have continued to be "In the Mode," which means the daily application of a minimum of 12% freshly-activated Vitamin C followed by 5% natural Vitamin E. All it takes is 2 steps in 2 minutes 2 times a day, and being mindful of how easy it is to oxidize.

The Evolution of Malibu Wellness

The success of my results after my accident, along with the research by biologists and chemists on the topical application of fresh-dried vitamins, led us to create C-Free Enterprises in

1985, organized exclusively for the purpose of using Vitamin C topically on the human body. It took awhile to convince the medical and salon industries to discover that we could solve problems for them that no other products could, just by using Vitamin C. Many of the solutions were immediate, while some took a week or sometimes a month, but hair, skin and scalp problems were being solved using the L-ascorbic acid form of Vitamin C along with natural Vitamin E.

One of our brands is Malibu 2000. Since everyone was calling and asking for "Malibu," we took the emphasis off "Vitamin C" and changed our name to Malibu Wellness, Inc. However, our mission has remained the same. At our Wellness Institute in Malibu, hair and skin care professionals are taught Total Oxidation Management so they can pass along these benefits to their respective clients and patients. Our education at the Institute and on our web site, www.WellnessSalon.com, continues to be centered around Vitamin C and Vitamin E and the relationship between those vitamins, our skin and the environment.

Knowledge is Power

Your desire to learn more about the simple science of skin by reading "You're Not Aging, You're Just Oxidizing" will empower you to make better decisions about what skin care products you purchase, what skin services you allow by a professional, and what lifestyle choices you make to slow your aging process.

By making the lifestyle changes suggested in this book, you can begin to slow the signs of aging and at the same time, normalize many abnormal skin conditions.

Chapter 2

TOTAL OXIDATION MANAGEMENT

Aging Assumptions

Most of us have looked in the mirror and realized that what we once thought of as "growing up" has turned into "growing older." The visible signs of aging begin to show, and most of us assume there is nothing we can do about it. While aging is a fact of life, you have more control over it than you might think.

You can learn how to slow the *process* of aging. The key word is "process," and you can manage many of the conditions that determine how fast you will age. The aging process is better understood today than just a few years ago. Most credit for this new awareness should go to researcher and doctor, Denham Harman, M.D.

Harman's Theory of Aging

Denham Harman's more than 50 years of study has shown that the major cause of aging is the action of oxygen that causes free radicals. Harman discovered that free radical reactions, however initiated, could be responsible for the progressive deterioration of biological systems over time because of their inherent ability to produce random change and destruction.

Harman theorized that an average person could live to within one to three years of the life expectancy of 85 by maintaining a healthy weight and eating foods adequate in essential nutrients. Harman believed that eating a lot of fruits and vegetables minimizes free radical reactions in the body.

As we age, however, diet alone is not enough to provide the adequate amount of antioxidants needed to slow the aging process. Harman believes that supplements are critical–especially vitamins C and E–while minimizing the accumulation of metals such as iron, copper and manganese, which are capable of initiating adverse free radical reactions.

In addition to Harman's theory, many older theories exist about what causes the signs of aging. Most of them in modern times have centered on two central themes: Genetics and Environment.

Genetics & Environment

While often discussed independently from each other, research shows genetics and environment are interconnected. These two theories alone do not provide an explanation of *why* we age. They can, however, contribute to our understanding of *how fast* we age.

Genetics and environment, along with lifestyle choices, are *conditions* that contribute to aging, but are not the *causes*. You can't escape genetics, and you are stuck with the environment of the city or town in which you've chosen to live. But that doesn't mean you can't do something about the effect these conditions have on your skin. The exciting news is that you can slow the aging process no matter what your skin color and no matter where you live.

Intrinsic vs. Extrinsic Factors that Contribute to Aging

Two classifications of aging exist: *intrinsic* or *extrinsic.* When something is described as intrinsic, it implies something that we cannot change, such as the color of our skin. Something that is extrinsic implies we have the power to do something to change it, such as choosing not to stay out in the sun without protection.

Intrinsic factors include those that will not change no matter what you do. The environment we live in is intrinsic since we can't change the climate. Another example is that many believe there is a clock ticking, and our cells that are programmed to break down at a certain age will do so due to genetics.

For example, the number of reproductive eggs a woman is born with is usually thought to be intrinsic. Women typically can release fertilizable eggs from the time of puberty until their late 40s or early 50s. After that time, their ovaries stop releasing eggs. That is intrinsically predetermined and lifestyle does not seem to make a difference.

Extrinsic signs of aging are those that appear only when you are exposed to external conditions, and you have the power to control how much you are exposed to those conditions that are causing you to age faster. How soon we show signs of aging is dependent upon our lifestyle choices – therefore we can control these factors.

Many consider lines around the mouth as intrinsic. However, they are often extrinsic because they wouldn't exist unless something triggers it, such as cigarettes, which are known to cause lines to form. The constant "puckering" smokers do to inhale uses tiny muscles in the face that over time oxidize, since free radicals are formed from the direct contact of the exhaled smoke. This constant pattern of behavior over a long period of time forms the lines, which are caused by oxidation.

Think of body builders who squint when they lift heavy weights. Over time, these "squints" become lines and wrinkles depending upon other conditions in their environment that affect their oxidation. There are many other examples, from squinting on a sunny day to "smile" lines.

Genetics: The Cards You Were Dealt

Before you assume that your skin is the way it is because of your parents' skin, think again. You do not have to show the same signs of aging as your parents. Of course, if you are 70, there is less chance for you to make some of the necessary changes than if you are 18. However, if you are a parent with a young child, you can raise your child to age more slowly by teaching a lifestyle of moderation through Total Oxidation Management. Then, your child will have a *reason* not to smoke and will have a *reason* not to go into a tanning bed. Most times, all we need is a reason to change our behavior because we now understand why we should do something differently.

But what about the color of your skin, which is one of the most important aspects of aging? It is true that the darker your skin and hair, the slower your skin and hair will age or oxidize. This also infers that the fairer your skin and hair, the faster they will oxidize—but only if you don't manage your oxidation. If you are fair skinned, the more Total Oxidation Management is important to you. The more pigment you have in your skin, the more natural Total Oxidation Management you already have built in.

Environment: The World Around You

Where you live and how long you have lived there, along with the choices you've made, have already affected your aging process. Your "environment" can be as broad as how warm or cold it is in the city or town you've chosen to live, or as narrow as the water you use to bathe in every day.

The good news is that we don't have to move or change work environments to have control over how fast we age. Once you understand the factors in the environment that effect aging, you can begin to take control and manage those factors.

The three environmental factors which have the most consequences on how you age are:

1. Air
2. Water
3. Sun

These factors and how they accelerate your aging process are explained in further detail in later chapters.

You Do Have Control Over Some Intrinsic Factors

Abnormal conditions of the skin, such as dandruff, eczema, and psoriasis have been considered intrinsic, usually linked genetically to others in the family who suffer the same conditions. I am a good example of how an intrinsic condition such as eczema can be changed—I can do something about it because I know that certain water and some shampoos trigger my eczema as a response to the external conditions. I use Total Oxidation Management to control the conditions that trigger my eczema. Therefore, I believe that some eczema and dandruff can be regarded as extrinsic because I can do something about them.

In my opinion, many signs of aging that have been thought to be intrinsic are in fact extrinsic. In other words, you can do something about them. For example, you have tiny muscles in your face that experience atrophy over the years: this could be categorized as an intrinsic form of aging. When your muscles lose their inherent tone, they become relaxed and the skin that covers them becomes "droopy." But we know that if we strengthen a muscle, it continues to be toned. So, even though muscle atrophy is intrinsic, the fact we can do something about it is extrinsic, since we can strengthen our muscles to keep the skin more toned, preventing some of the signs of aging.

Wrinkles were considered to be intrinsic until just a few years ago, and many people still believe they will wrinkle just like their parents did. Now, it is well known that most of the breakdown of cells is due to free radicals caused by some kind of oxidation. It could be the breakdown is occurring from some kind of internal oxidation activity. However, as we learn more and more about how oxidation occurs and how to manage free radicals, we don't have to accept that wrinkles are inevitable, "no matter what I do."

Learning a New Vocabulary

"Oxidation" and "free radicals" are foreign words to many. Strangely enough, people are using the word "antioxidant" as if they completely understand the meaning. However, until you have an understanding of oxidation, you cannot fully understand antioxidants—you will learn even more about these terms in later chapters.

Simply put, if oxidation is anything that speeds up the addition of oxygen (such as water, sun or air) to something else (skin, for example), then an "antioxidant" is a substance that prevents the speeding up of oxidation. An antioxidant changes the molecular structure of an oxidizer and stops the oxidation process. A key element of Total Oxidation Management is the external application of antioxidants Vitamin C and Vitamin E, which are more fully explained in following chapters.

Once you understand what an antioxidant is and how it can affect your skin, you will be better prepared to ask some important questions about all the products that claim to have antioxidant benefits. More importantly, you can begin to see new relationships between your environment and your external body. You will be able to talk to your skin care specialist and discuss options for the care of your skin. Most importantly, you will be in charge of yourself and not be dependent on someone else for all your answers. You have the opportunity to manage how fast you show the signs of aging once you understand oxidative free radicals, where they are, and how they affect you.

Managing Oxidation is Simple

Skin is our cover, our great protector, our armor. The trade-off for the protection skin provides our bodies is the constant wear and tear it endures. Skin has a memory and shows signs of past battles, and can wear down and lose much of its ability to defend us as we age.

The older we get, the slower the rate of our skin's exfoliation, and the more important it is to help normalize the reproduction of skin cells by increasing collagen development and keratin protein synthesis. As we age, we must strive to maintain as much of the "normal" conditions our bodies experienced when we were younger and healthier and when we had less wear and tear on our skin.

Progressive research in the past two decades has led to much more confidence in determining how fast skin will show signs of aging. Once you understand the primary oxidation that causes cell damage, you can determine what damage you have probably already done, can prevent future damage, and reverse some existing damage. Most exciting is that you will learn how easy it is to manage the oxidation on your skin.

Are You Making Assumptions that Might Cause You to Appear to Age Faster?

*The number one cause of the aging
of skin is genetics.*   *True*   *False*

*Your skin will age at about the same
rate as your parents.*   *True*   *False*

*A chemical peel will slow oxidation
and help prevent free radicals.*   *True*   *False*

*Someone who has a tanned-looking
face has at least some skin damage.*   *True*   *False*

*Chlorine in a pool can age skin,
but the chlorine in your shower
does not age skin.*   *True*   *False*

*Skin care products with antioxidants
on the label will slow aging.*   *True*   *False*

*A sunscreen with a SPF 45 will block
all the rays that can lead
to premature aging.*   *True*   *False*

*Exercise is a sure way to slow the
visible signs of aging.*   *True*   *False*

*New Oxygen therapies for skin will
prevent wrinkles, age spots and
other signs of aging.*   *True*   *False*

*Signs of aging caused by cigarettes
are irreversible.*   *True*   *False*

All the statements above are false. On the next page is a
short explanation of why each is false.

Answering Your Assumptions

The number one cause of the aging of skin is genetics. False

The number one cause of aging is oxidation. Genetics does not cause aging, even though it does play a significant role in how fast you oxidize, or show signs of aging. The pigment or lack of pigment can affect how fast your skin oxidizes.

Your skin will age at about the same rate as your parents. False

The only reason your skin will age as your parents is your environment and lifestyle conditions are similar and you did little or nothing to prevent the aging process (oxidation) from occurring.

A chemical peel will slow oxidation and help prevent free radicals. False

A skin peel that removes protective layers of skin does nothing to stop or slow the process of oxidation or aging. A chemical peel might leave your skin free of wrinkles and age spots for the short term, but the exposure to oxidation following the process can be much more damaging than any of the short term benefits that are achieved.

Someone who has a tanned-looking face has at least some skin damage. False

Skin cells that are tanned from exposure to any UV rays have at least some damage to his or her skin. However, if the tanned appearance is the result of a bronzer or self-tanner lotion or spray chemical such as DHA sugar that can stain the skin a caramelized color, it can actually help protect the skin from oxidation and slow the aging process.

**Chlorine in a pool can age skin,
but the chlorine in your shower
does not age skin.**   **False**

The amount of chlorine now being used in water systems
in most communities is higher than is legally required in
swimming pools, and actually causes the skin to oxidize
faster , triggering free radicals to form that can in turn lead
to an acceleration of the appearance of signs of aging.

**Skin care products with "antioxidants"
on the label will slow aging.**   **False**

Just because a product claims to include one or several antioxidants provides you no guarantees that these ingredients
have any benefit to slowing the aging of the skin. I would
estimate that of the majority of skin care products that claim
to include antioxidants for prevention of aging have little or
no benefits. The FDA does not presently monitor effective
topical use of antioxidants; therefore, without knowing the
correct activity, percentage, delivery system and form, the
benefits of the antioxidant cannot be guaranteed.

**A sunscreen with a SPF 45 will block
all the rays that can lead
to premature aging.**   **False**

The FDA has clearly stated that no SPF blocks all damaging
UV rays and therefore any SPF will still allow some UV rays
to affect skin cells. Use of at least SPF 15 along with stable
Vitamin C and Vitamin E can broaden the scope of protection. Also, there is a concern that excess use of ingredients
in sunscreens of SPF 30 or more could be irritating to the
skin.

**Exercise is a sure way to slow the
visible signs of aging.**   **False**

Many forms of exercise have benefits that can slow signs of
aging; however, many forms of exercise will actually con-

tribute to accelerated signs of aging. Swimming, tennis, and golf enthusiasts who are exposed to oxidizers and sun show signs of aging often faster than the sedentary person who remains indoors.

New oxygen therapies for skin will prevent wrinkles, age spots and other signs of aging. **False**

More controversy than conclusive evidence exists that infusing oxygen topically, especially using oxidizers such as hydrogen peroxide, can help in any way to remove wrinkles, age spots and other signs of aging.

Signs of aging caused by cigarettes are irreversible. **False**

Regular use of freshly activated vitamins in the correct percentage, pH, and delivery system can absolutely result in the reversal of the appearance of fine lines caused by cigarettes.

Chapter 3

TOM
TOTAL OXIDATION MANAGEMENT

The Root of Oxidation

Putting the Brakes on Aging

To fully understand the premise of this book—which is that most signs of aging are the result of oxidation—you must first have an understanding of how oxidation works. The root of the word oxidation is "oxygen." You probably know that the chemical sign for oxygen is the letter "O." For example, H_2O is the sign for water and demonstrates there is one atom of O, which is Oxygen, in one molecule of water.

Oxygen is a primary component for the fuel of life—necessary for most of the energy created in our bodies and in our environment. Oxygen interacts with objects, plants and animals — including humans. This interaction usually involves air, sun, water, soil and/or chemicals—the very essential elements of life. However, *too* much of these good things will change the very structure of your skin's physical properties.

Oxygen: Our "Dangerous Friend"

Oxygen has been called our "dangerous friend" by one of the leading and most significant researchers of aging, Dr. Lester Packer, PhD from the University of California at Berkley. His research has led to a better understanding of the aging process and confirms the need for Total Oxidation Management.

A single atom of oxygen itself is not such a harmful radical. However, the metabolism of oxygen molecules (more than one atom) can produce by-products, called "oxygen free radicals" that in turn multiply, setting off a chain of damaging reactions. This damage is at the molecular and cellular levels and rather than being overtly toxic, it is slowly expressed as accelerated signs of aging and can lead to diseases, even cancer.

How Oxidation Leads to the Death of a Cell

Oxidation is action, a process. Visualize oxidation as the tiniest little spark. This spark is the action oxygen has on any substance that alters its molecular structure. Most oxidation is invisible when the process actually occurs; however, the results, even months or years later, are often very visible. And the visible signs of oxidation on skin are characterized as aging.

Accelerated oxidation leads to the formation of free radicals that will wreak havoc, causing damage on your skin. The good news is that stable, active antioxidant Vitamin C and Vitamin E can help normalize a free radical by donating an electron, creating a healthy pair of electrons bonding the atoms together to return a free radical back to a healthy molecule—no longer free to roam, free to destroy—it is back in its proper order and functions to contribute to your health.

With Total Oxidation Management, you can actually put the "brakes" on the free radicals that can create wrinkles, age spots, scars, sagging skin, and other signs of aging. Free radicals can occur whenever you're exposed to air, sun and water, and once you discover how it occurs, you can control how much damage is done.

Oxidation with Air, Sun & Water

The first thing many people associate with oxidation is rust on iron. When air, sun and water actually oxidize iron, the process is not visible. Over time, rust is formed, the visible result of the millions of invisible "tiny sparks" occurring when the air, sun and water constantly cause oxidation of iron. The rust on a car bumper or bicycle rim is oxidation. When you notice that the paint color on your car has faded, once again, you can blame oxidation.

Another example is the Statue of Liberty, which is made of copper. As it oxidized, it turned green, and that's how we view the Statue of Liberty today…as oxidized copper. Metals oxidize faster than most other substances, as they possess electrons that cause more ion or electrical activity as metals interact with our environment.

If oxidation can have a dramatic effect on a surface as tough and durable as the metals that make up cars and bicycles, imagine what oxidation can do to your external body—your skin, your scalp and your hair.

A friend recently told me that her mother would not drink one drop of water directly from the tap because she did not want to "rust" her insides. She brewed tea and other drinks that she professed would not cause her to rust…or oxidize. She was not so far off from reality. And today, the amount of oxidizing chlorine that is put into your community's drinking water adds credence to her claim.

Obviously, drinking water is important to promote healthy cells. To remove the active chlorine, sprinkle in a dash of fresh-dried ascorbic acid Vitamin C in each glass of water you drink.

However, water alone with one atom of oxygen does not significantly accelerate the process of oxidation, causing signs of aging. Still, some of the most damaging oxidation occurs *in conjunction* with water and sun.

Bleach is Oxidation

Bleach actually refers to many different processes of oxidation. You know that when you go outside and bleach your hair you are trying to lighten it with the combination of air (nitrogen and oxygen), water (hydrogen and oxygen), and sun (heat energy with oxygen).

We use the same word "bleach" for a chemical solution using chlorine or chloride to lighten your clothes. When you have your hair bleached at the salon, peroxide chemicals are used to bleach the hair to change the color.

Isn't it strange that we refer to the word "bleach" for all these processes when in reality, completely different sources are used to accomplish a similar bleaching effect? But what they each have in common is the fact that each process is all about – oxidizing! So when you use the word bleach, you are actually referring to "oxidation."

Play & Exercise—Oxidize!

You make a concerted effort to keep playing and exercising to stay young. But could it inadvertently be aging you? Outdoor sports, such as golf and tennis, are intended to keep you young; however, these healthy sports can actually cause visible signs of aging if your skin is not protected against harsh sun, wind, and water.

Swimmers, for example, receive excellent health benefits from their exercise, but they need to understand that they might be the most oxidized of all athletes due to the harsh effects of chlorine, water, and sun on their hair and skin. Just look at a master swimmer–their skin is oxidized even though their muscle tone and flexibility is usually in excellent condition.

There are two ways exercise speeds up oxidation. First, the exposure of the skin to oxidizing environments can increase the aging process. Second, the metabolism of the oxygen during exercise can increase the number of free radicals that are formed. Proper nutrition and recommended supplements can help keep both the vitamins and necessary enzymes at levels that can offset the formation and spreading of internal free radicals.

I am not saying don't exercise, rather, make sure you protect yourself with Total Oxidation Management when you do.

Fortunately, by understanding Total Oxidation Management and the use of fresh-dried Vitamin C and natural Vitamin E, the swimmer, golfer, and tennis player can dramatically improve their skin and hair conditions, and slow the process of aging.

Defensive and offensive Total Oxidation Management becomes as important as the defense and offense of the game itself. Take a closer look at your activities, the environment, and the exposure to the chemicals around you to determine if your attempt to slow the aging process is actually speeding up your aging process. Plus, not only is your outdoor environment aging you, your inside environment can be, too.

How Your Home & Work Can be Oxidizing Environments

You could be speeding up your oxidation just taking a shower or going to work every day. Do you live or work in an environment that speeds up oxidation? As you read through the later chapters, consider what might be hiding in the air, the water, or the conditions around you that could slowly, over time, increase how much and how fast your skin is oxidized. We all live in an oxidizing environment; once we understand the oxidizers we are exposed to, we can shift our lifestyle to adapt and manage it.

How Fast is Your Skin Oxidizing

Test how you compare your potential for aging against others. Respond once to each of the seven questions below and total your scores to determine how fast you might show signs of aging.

1. What is your skin type?

____Very Dark	2
____Dark	4
____Medium	8
____Fair	12
____Very fair	14

2. What is the color of your eyes?

___Dark Brown	2
___Light Brown	3
___Green	4
___Blue	5

3. What is (was) the natural color of your hair?

___Black	0
___Dark Brown	1
___Brown	2
___Light Brown	3
___Blonde	4
___Red	5

4. Exposure to sun.

___Never tanned or burned	0
___Tanned seldom but never sunburned	4
___Tanned often and sunburned at least once	8
___Tanned and/or sunburned numerous times	10

5. Exposure to tanning bed.

____Less than 12 sessions ever	2
____12 – 24 sessions ever	4
____25-35 sessions ever	6
____36 – 45 sessions ever	8
____over 45 sessions ever	10

6. Exposure to cigarette smoke.

____Never smoked	0
____Smoked less than 5 years	5
____Smoked 5 - 10 years	10
____Smoked 10 - 20 years	15
____Smoked more than 20 years	20

7. Exposure to pollution.

____Never lived in an air-polluted area	0
____Lived in an air-polluted area less than 5 years	2
____Lived in an air-polluted area for more than 5 years	4

TOTAL

____**Add your scores to determine your potential for oxidized, aged skin.**

Score Summary

Under 25:	Will slowly show signs of aging.
25- 35:	Will moderately show signs of aging.
Over 36:	Will rapidly show signs of aging.

Chapter 4

TOM

TOTAL OXIDATION MANAGEMENT

The "Cost" of Free Radicals

Now you know that the most significant cause of aging, skin disorders and many skin diseases is oxidation. Oxidation creates free radicals, and free radicals damage healthy cells. Therefore, the most important maintenance for skin is to protect healthy cells from becoming oxidized, and to help normalize existing free radicals to prevent them from spreading—which is the objective of Total Oxidation Management.

Some of the most obvious forms of oxidation in our environment include exposure to the sun's UV rays, tanning beds, pollution exposure, chlorinated water, and cigarette smoke. But since skin is constantly exposed to these elements, it remains a prime target for oxidation and free radical damage. A clear understanding of what free radicals are will help you minimize the effects they have on your skin.

A Closer Look at Free Radicals

Free radicals are unstable atoms and molecules. They are so radical in their destruction that they can change DNA codes to produce mutations, creating newly formed cells that are foreign to the body, and can eventually lead to tumors and skin cancer.

A single free radical is not a serious issue until it attacks other healthy molecules, creating a chain of events that progressively leads to thousands, millions, and even trillions of free radicals within the skin and in the body.

Free Radicals: Unattached Atoms in Search of Electrons

All substances are made up of millions of tiny atoms. These atoms form small groups called "molecules" that together form "cells." Within each healthy molecule, atoms are bonded together by pairs of electrons. These pairs of electrons act to hold the atoms together in their proper order. If these atoms remain stable, someone ages slowly. If the atoms are not in pairs, the cells they make up are damaged and even destroyed, speeding up the aging process.

Accelerated oxidation is much like a spark causing something to combust. When oxidation occurs, one or more of the atoms can lose an electron, changing a healthy functioning molecule into a damaging free radical.

In an attempt to gain an electron to replace the missing electron, this free radical "steals" an electron from an otherwise healthy pair, which are already bonding healthy atoms together. The sad reality is that a free radical can steal an electron from a healthy molecule and create more free radicals—but the electron that was stolen cannot necessarily even be used by the original free radical. Now rather than just "trading even," we have free radicals creating more free radicals just trying to get normalized and healthy again.

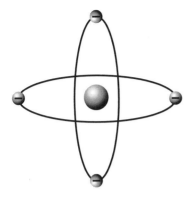

Stable Atom
Even number of electrons.

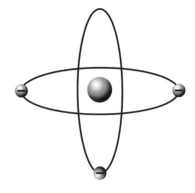

Unstable Atom (Free Radical)
1 electron is missing.

Remember that when free radicals exist and begin to steal electrons from healthy molecules, they can multiply, and even cause changes in the DNA structure of the cell. This spreading of free radicals can eventually cause mutations that can lead to the development of tumors, leading to the formation of various forms of cancer. Therefore, a lifestyle of Total Oxidation Management not only can slow your aging process, but it also might prevent an early death.

The Slow Destroyer, Inside and Out

Oxidizing free radicals are not like a fast-acting lethal poison. They are more like a slow, often unnoticed evil force. Free radicals occur one at a time, unless you are exposed to a sudden high dose of oxidation. Bleach, sunburn, and radiation therapies are three examples of accelerated free radical production. Otherwise, free radical damage usually occurs over a long period of time by continuously multiplying, leading to signs of aging. This is the reason you need to be very aware of your lifestyle patterns and determine those that increase oxidation and those that can help manage oxidation.

Probably the fastest production of free radicals that you have experienced personally is sunburn, since sunburn is inflammation resulting from the formation of free radicals. As you know, the intensity is much worse the second day than on the day of the burn. That is the continuation of free radicals spreading, causing more free radicals to form.

On the other hand, cigarettes are often characterized as the slow "silent killer," because the formation of free radicals and the oxidative damage to the lungs occurs over a long period of time. If only an alarm would sound every time a molecule becomes a free radical, a smoker would be more aware of potential damage, and Total Oxidation Management would be even simpler to accomplish.

A good example of someone excessively oxidizing themselves without being aware of it occurred following a class I taught at a very impressive beauty school in Ventura County, Calif. A very nice young woman stopped me in the parking lot to ask me some questions. As I was listening to her, I noticed that her face was extremely red with inflammation. I asked her if she recently had a chemical peel, and she replied that she just had her second chemical peel in the past two months.

As we were standing in the hot sun, I became aware of her facial skin that should not have had even minutes of sun exposure. And then, within seconds, she pulled her cigarette from behind her back to light up. I watched the smoke smother her face. I began to visualize the tiny little sparks of oxidation that were creating trillions of free radicals on her exposed, unprotected, newly developing skin cells. Any benefits she thought she had received from the peel just "went up in smoke." She will likely see severe damage in months or years to come.

This is an example of extreme oxidation. For most of us, however, day-to-day oxidation is subtler, and free radicals form more slowly, accumulating as we age. The good news is that oxidation is a process that can be managed to improve the way we look and feel: Total Oxidation Management of the environment around us.

Oxygen: A Necessary Evil

Oxidation is an on-going important and necessary energy producing process inside our bodies. Over a thousand free radicals are formed every day. The by-products created by the metabolism of oxygen in the mitochondria, the energy factories of our cells, are free radicals. They are much like exaust pollution that is the by-product of cars when gas is converted to energy.

The key word is "by-product." The free radical is the waste that occurs when cells are affected and energy is produced. Internally, vitamins, along with important enzymes, work to normalize free radicals. When researchers can guarantee effectiveness of enzymes such as SOD (superoxide dismutase) can be replicated or extracted for external therapies, we might see another chapter of anti-aging opportunities.

Now that you have a vision of what a free radical is, you can better understand how to stop, slow or at least defend every skin cell against the formation of free radicals with Total Oxidation Management. This can be accomplished by either blocking the exposure to oxidizers or by using ingredients such as the fresh-dried L-ascorbic acid form of Vitamin C and natural Vitamin E to help normalize the free radicals when they occur.

Chapter

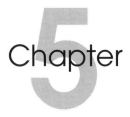

TOM
TOTAL OXIDATION MANAGEMENT

Vitamin C & Vitamin E
are Superior

Start Fighting the Signs of Aging Today

The use of the right vitamins on your skin—in the correct percentages, in the correct pH and in an effective delivery system—can change your life, or at least how you look and feel. While other chemicals and minerals have demonstrated some value to skin, nothing has as far reaching benefits as the topical application of the L-ascorbic acid form of Vitamin C followed by natural Vitamin E. This is the essence of Total Oxidation Management.

The past decade has been a free-for-all on claims and marketing hype regarding vitamins, fruit acids, extracts and other naturally derived ingredients proclaiming to be the new fountain of youth. When I first learned about some of the benefits of Vitamin C and Vitamin E in the early 80's, my first reaction was "Oh, sure, vitamins can cure the common cold and now conditions of the skin." It took only a few simple demonstrations with oxidizers for me to understand the powerful and important role these two antioxidant vitamins play—especially Vitamin C. First, following is an explanation of vitamins and their role in managing oxidation.

Vitamins: Vita=Vital—It's Life!

The Polish chemist, Casimir Funk conceived the word "vitamin" in 1912, defining a category for substances that are necessary to sustain life.

In the United States, thirteen vitamins are recognized as "vital." It is important to realize that vitamins are not found in the body naturally and do not produce energy. However, vitamins do often help in the conversion of food into energy. Vitamins must be consumed either through foods or supplements, or synthesized by an external source (e.g. the sun's ability to be a catalyst for Vitamin D to be produced in the skin and travel through the body, and some Vitamin B's are metabolized in the intestines).

Another example of a vitamin created by an external source is the new Vitamin F, which is composed of two fatty acids— linoleic acid (LA) and alpha-linoleic acid (LNA). There are two basic categories of essential fatty acids—Omega-3 and Omega-6—which the body is not capable of manufacturing. In Europe, Vitamin F is recognized as a vitamin, but not yet in the U.S. until the Recommended Daily Allowance has been determined by the FDA.

An important contributor to the field of internal and external vitamins is David Djerassi, director of the Specialty and Cosmetic Chemicals Group of Roche Vitamins, Inc. (now DSM Nutritionals). For over two decades, Djerassi made it clear that no one vitamin is the exclusive answer to all of our needs. His leadership in the area of vitamin research has resulted in many companies, such as ours, that have continued to discover new uses and new contributions of vitamins to the human body.

Cells Absorb Vitamins: Water vs. Oil

Cells in our body—and most importantly, our skin—are categorized as either water cells or oil (fat/lipid) cells. Therefore, an ingredient or product compound must be either water and/ or oil soluble to be absorbed and positively affect a cell.

All vitamins are either water-soluble or oil-(fat/lipid) soluble. Water-soluble vitamins are vitamins that are absorbed, stored, or effective in water cells. Fat soluble vitamins are vitamins absorbed, stored, or effective in oil cells. Of course, most of our skin is made up of water cells, but fat cells are also very important in providing defensive skin functions. This is the reason it is important to include both water-soluble and fat- soluble vitamins in your daily skin care.

The following chart divides the different vitamins (including Omega III Vitamin F) by water or oil solubility to help you understand this important aspect of vitamins:

Water Soluble Vitamins	Oil (Fat/Lipid) Soluble Vitamins
Vitamin C	Vitamin A
Vitamin B1 (thiamin)	Vitamin D
Vitamin B2(riboflavin)	Vitamin E
Vitamin B3 (niacin)	Vitamin K
Vitamin B5 (including panthenol pro-vitamin B5)	Vitamin F * (Omega III Fats)
Vitamin B6 (pyroxidine)	
Vitamin B12 (Cobalamin)	
Folic acid (a B vitamin sometimes called vitamin H)	
Biotin (a B vitamin)	

*Not yet a vitamin in the U.S.

The reason that the L-ascorbic acid form of Vitamin C is such an important vitamin is that it is so versatile and is water-soluble; important, because approximately 70% of our skin is comprised of water. Ascorbic acid is the form of Vitamin C that the body most readily recognizes, and even if other forms of Vitamin C are ingested or applied, the body still must convert those forms back to ascorbic acid to reap the benefits.

Vitamin E is oil soluble and therefore absorbed by oil/fat/ lipid cells. Vitamin E acetate is the form that is used most often externally because it is easily absorbed by skin and creates a smooth skin texture and helps heal wounds. Most Vitamin E is produced synthetically, but now, natural Vitamin E has become available, with clinical studies suggesting it is more effective than synthetic Vitamin E.

Marketing Hype vs. Clinical Studies

In the past ten years, how many times have you read or seen an ad that sounded too good to be true? And it was not until you tried the product, that you realized the marketing hype around it.

Learning to "read between the lines" is essential in order for you to understand the ingredients on the labels of the products you purchase. Because vitamin technology is still relatively new and the standards are not established for claims regarding vitamins, consumers need to take charge of their own "Total Oxidation Management."

For instance, not all the vitamins listed above have been found to benefit the external body. My research suggests these vitamins can be categorized into four groups as they relate to our hair, scalp and skin:

1) Important

2) Beneficial

3) Potentially Beneficial

4) Unnecessary

The following chart indicates the value for the external application of vitamins.

Important	Beneficial	Potentially Beneficial	Benefits Less Clear or Unknown
Vitamin C	Vitamin A	Vitamin D	B1 Thiamin
Vitamin E	Vitamin B3 Niacin	Vitamin F	B6 Pyroxidine
	Vitamin B5 Pantothenic (Panthenol)	Vitamin K	B12 Cobalamin
	Vitamin H Biotin (B complex)	Vitamin B2 Riboflavin	

As you'll notice from the chart above, two of the most important vitamins for external application are Vitamin C and Vitamin E, both antioxidants.

Understanding the Word Antioxidant

"Antioxidant" is the most abused word in personal care. If oxidation is the primary cause of damage to our skin, then "anti-oxidation" is something that has the ability to stop or prevent that destructive wearing down of our outer covering. Antioxidant vitamins are essential in protecting the epidermis from damage by free radicals. Antioxidants decrease this damage and can contribute to health and longevity. Most scientists agree that antioxidant supplementation is a valuable means for slowing down and preventing premature aging.

The word "antioxidant," as with so many marketing buzzwords, has been used and abused to the point it has assumptions associated with it that are just not true. When we began introducing fresh-dried antioxidants in hair, scalp and skin care 18 years ago, we were unaware of any competing personal care manufacturer using them. In 1985, under the name of C-Free (Chlorine Free, Chemical Free with Vitamin

C), we began teaching professionals about antioxidants. However, many people could not understand why we would use a word that began with such a negative prefix: "anti." It was not until the early 1990's that the word antioxidant became more widely used, even though most consumers now think they have heard of antioxidants all their life. The fact is, antioxidants are still a relatively new concept which needs further understanding by both professionals and consumers.

In fact, I remember talking to a prestigious plastic surgeon about antioxidants in skin care products. He commented that he assumed that if the product said it had antioxidants and was sold through the professional skin and hair care industries, it had met a specific standard, suggesting that most antioxidant products are equally effective.

This is not true.

Antioxidants are Not Created Equal

Antioxidants all have some ability to alter some form of oxidation to make it less damaging. By donating an electron to a free radical, an antioxidant can help normalize an unhealthy molecule that could have led to an unhealthy cell. However, just because something is an antioxidant in the lab, does not necessarily make it effective in a product for the skin and hair. The variables that determine the effectiveness of an antioxidant element or compound are the:

1) Specific chemical structure of the antioxidant.

2) Stability of the activity of the antioxidant.

3) Compatibility of the antioxidant to the structure of the skin and hair.

4) Ability for the antioxidant to penetrate the skin and hair surface.

5) Amount and/or percentage of the antioxidant in the product.

The Right Antioxidants Work

Earlier, we discussed how free radicals are formed from oxidation. Remember that the damage is done when an electron is lost in the pair bonding atoms together.

Think of a superior, active antioxidant as a type of "free radical fixer," able to help improve the appearance of lines and wrinkles and prevent free radicals from damaging cells. Furthermore, research is clear that antioxidants are often more effective when used in conjunction with other antioxidants, suggesting there is significant advantages to using vitamins that are interconnected in their actions.

The research that confirmed my confidence in the use of externally applied antioxidant vitamins was the research conducted at Ball State University by Dr. Keith Ault and at the University of Illinois by Dr. Joseph Larson. Their findings suggest that the body transports any available Vitamin C through the sweat to the surface layers of the skin, convincing me that the body uses Vitamin C externally to provide both protection and performance of healthier cells—confirming that applying antioxidants such as Vitamin C topically to our skin is imperative to managing oxidation. Since that early research, hundreds of clinical studies have confirmed the significant effects of Vitamin C in and on the skin.

Vitamin C is a Superior Antioxidant

The L-ascorbic acid form of Vitamin C is the most versatile antioxidant vitamin because it provides so many different benefits all at the same time. Knowing the body extracts Vitamin C from foods and supplements taken internally and transports any available vitamin to the external skin layers and out of the body through sweat is the foundation of what we teach professionals at the Malibu Wellness Institute.

It is clear that nature has a specific intent for using Vitamin C externally for protection and performance of cellular activity in the skin and ultimately, even the scalp and hair. And since most people do not ingest enough food containing adequate Vitamin C, and the environment in which we live is more oxidizing than ever, supplementing the L-ascorbic form of Vitamin C directly on the skin is a necessity for healthier cells.

When we began using Vitamin C externally in 1985, very little research had been conducted in the U.S. to help confirm or contradict what we were learning on the thousands of people who were using our Vitamin C. Most of the early research came from Europe, as well as from David Djerassi, who encouraged our use of various forms of Vitamin C—including L-ascorbic acid, ascorbyl palmatate, and new variations that continued to become available...but still, none are superior to ascorbic acid.

I learned later that years after we began selling products using Vitamin C for the external body, studies in the late 1980's and early 90's by researchers at major universities—including Duke University and the University of Wisconsin—were being conducted confirming new applications for Vitamin C. Those whose research on Vitamin C are regarded as the most important and significant beyond that of David Djerassi include Dr. Sheldon Pinnell and Dr. David Darr. Their research, along with ongoing studies on oxidation, free radicals, and aging of skin, has brought Malibu Wellness' use of Vitamin C from a limited group of professionals to a world of consumers now seeking the truth in Vitamin C.

Confusion Regarding Various Forms of Vitamin C

Raw ingredient suppliers have worked to expand the availability of newer forms of Vitamin C. Some of these forms include sodium ascorbate, coated encapsulated Vitamin C (liposomes & nanosomes), magnesium ascorbyl phosphate and sodium ascorbyl phosphate. All of these newer forms are much more expensive and less effective than L-ascorbic acid, and it is important to remember that the form of Vitamin C the body most benefits from is ascorbic acid. And all of these compound forms of Vitamin C begin with the basic structure of L-ascorbic acid, which the body works to convert back into L-ascorbic acid to be used and metabolized by cells.

The abundance of Vitamin C in the cells of the deeper layers of the epidermis demonstrates the body's need for this versatile vitamin for healthy cell development and adequate functionality. Yet, since Vitamin C is used in both the offense and defense of healthy cell maintenance, the need for both an adequate intake of foods rich in Vitamin C along with the application of the vitamin is important to Total Oxidation Management.

Effective Use of Externally Applied Vitamin C

Eighteen years of research on the use of Vitamin C on humans has led me to conclude that in order for Vitamin C to be the most effective, it must be:

1) The ascorbic acid form of Vitamin C.

2) Active and stable.

3) Used in no less than an active 10% solution at the time of usage.

4) Formulated in an acid pH of 3.

1) L-Ascorbic Acid Form of Vitamin C – After years of testing various forms of Vitamin C, we have found that the L-ascorbic acid form of Vitamin C is the only form, or at least the most effective form, necessary to achieve numerous benefits. In 1986, we thought ascorbyl palmitate would be the best form, but soon we learned that it is not stable after about six months of being mixed in a skin or hair product. Ascorbyl palmitate is good if it is stable but it is not as effective and does not provide all the benefits of the freshly activated and stable ascorbic acid form of Vitamin C.

41

Other forms such as liposomes of coated Vitamin C are interesting, but very expensive and not superior to fresh-dried Vitamin C. In the past five years, sodium and magnesium ascorbyl phosphate have become available and they have been found to be stable for over a year after mixed in a product; however, it is very expensive and the pH of the product must be higher than the recommended, and more ideal, acid form. Additionally, I have never seen a product that uses a high enough concentration of these other forms of Vitamin C to feel confident it can deliver the benefits of the L-ascorbic acid form of Vitamin C. Some of the alternative forms of Vitamin C might provide some of the antioxidant qualities of L-ascorbic acid, but the L-ascorbic form of Vitamin C in the proper pH, concentration, and delivery system can be beneficial to the skin, scalp and hair beyond the antioxidant features.

2) Active and Stable – These are the most important issues surrounding the L-ascorbic acid form of Vitamin C. It is well known that once it is in any solution and exposed to heat—even room temperature—over a period of time the vitamin activity begins breaking down through approximately six stages until it becomes a sugar. Therefore, it is not that Vitamin C goes "bad;" it just loses its ability to provide its unique benefits. Therefore, any time you are seeking the true benefits of Vitamin C, be sure you or your professional freshly activates the Vitamin C in the products. And you will know if the vitamin is breaking down into a sugar because it will begin to turn from clear to yellow to brown. Store your freshly activated Vitamin C product in a cool, dark place.

3) Used in No Less Than a 10% Solution – A product label should include that product's percentage of Vitamin C, but few do. However, even if the percentage is declared on the label, if the product has already been activated in a solution prior to your purchasing it, you have no way of knowing the current percentage of Vitamin C in the solution. As noted above, Vitamin C goes through stages of breaking down into a sugar, and a product that might have included 20% active Vitamin C when it was manufactured very likely has 0% of Vitamin C by the time you purchase it. You are likely spending over $100 an ounce for sugar water.

4) Acid pH Around 3 – The benefits of the L-ascorbic form of Vitamin C are more than the antioxidant qualities. This unique vitamin when formulated with the correct pH can help normalize the exfoliation of the scalp and offset the alkaline ammonias that might be excreted from the skin if your internal pH is too acidic. Additionally, it can help keep your pores tight and your hair cuticle closed, giving you a smoother complexion and shinier hair.

Benefits of Vitamin C

People have often called the benefits that Vitamin C has on the external body a miracle. It is not a miracle. It is nature's approach to providing protection and performance to the essence of life. As we have discovered, Vitamin C is surrounding life at the point of reproduction (seeds, fetus, etc.); nature uses the vitamin for offense and defense, performance and protection. The exciting and incredible benefits of Vitamin C that have been demonstrated by thousands of users and/or through clinical research include:

1) Antioxidant Protection

2) Prevention of Photo-Aging

3) Normalizing of Skin Exfoliation

4) Inducing and Benefiting Collagen Synthesis

5) Slowing the Synthesis of Melanin

6) Reducing Inflammation

1) Antioxidant Protection - The use of the L-ascorbic acid form of Vitamin C as an antioxidant is probably the best known feature. The benefits include the ability to stop and prevent oxidizers from affecting the external body by scavenging free radicals and helping normalize otherwise damaged cells. These features and benefits are further explained throughout this book.

2) Prevention of Photo-Aging – The use of the L-ascorbic acid form of Vitamin C on the skin can prevent, and have been reported to remove, the formation of age spots, wrinkles, fine lines and other forms of photo-aging caused by free radicals resulting from exposure to sun and oxidizers. The ability of Vitamin C to donate an electron to a free radical can change the molecule from a damaged and destructive molecule to a healthy productive molecule.

3) Normalize Skin Exfoliation – Applied in a pH of 3, the L-ascorbic form of Vitamin C can help promote the natural synthesis of exfoliation rather than speed it up as done by AHA, glycolic acid, and other more radical exfoliation ingredients. This key feature of Vitamin C is important to many of the natural functions of the skin and hair proteins that play such an important role in our appearance and overall health of our skin. The contrast to chemical peels and other radical exfoliation issues are explained in later chapters.

4) Induce and Benefit Collagen Synthesis – The water retention of the collagen and elastin fibers is very important to the normal development and function in the dermis layer of skin. The depletion of this water-based gel matrix can increase the appearance of wrinkles while also causing the skin to be thinner with less elasticity. Since the L-ascorbic acid form of Vitamin C is water soluble, it plays an important role, as demonstrated in many in-vitro clinical studies, in the biosynthesis of collagen created by the fibroblasts factories deep in the skin. Vitamin C therefore helps increase and improve the strength and appearance of skin, especially in older men, as well as women after menopause when the synthesis of collagen otherwise slows down. This feature is a key to why Vitamin C is so beneficial in wound healing and in the basic repair of abnormal skin cells.

5) Slow the Synthesis of Melanin – In 1996, the *American Journal of Dermatology* reported research that suggested the use of the L-ascorbic form of Vitamin C slows the production of melanin that produces the pigment color to our skin. As the production of melanin occurs upon exposure to UV rays which cause oxidation free radicals, it is logical that the use of stable Vitamin C can help prevent the occurrence of excess pigment production of skin. This also explains some of the ability for this unique vitamin to help reduce signs of aging, such as age spots and freckles, that are the result of excess melanin in skin cells.

6) Reduce Skin Inflammation– The L-ascorbic acid form of Vitamin C has the ability to help suppress the inflammation of skin and accompanying side affects, such as redness. This appears to be a natural feature of how Vitamin C can help in nature's own response to the formation of free radicals. This can be especially beneficial in the appearance of conditions such as sunburn, rosacea, and physical or chemical burns.

Can you apply too much Vitamin C?

You can create what I call a "hyper C reaction" if you apply Vitamin C in too high a percentage and/or too low a pH. This is the reason we recommend a pH of approximately 3 in a solution of 12%. It works.

You can also use too much Vitamin C and get it on your clothes. If you do, it will caramelize and should be treated as a food-grade stain.

Partnered along side another powerful antioxidant, Vitamin C becomes even more beneficial.

Vitamin E: an Antioxidant Partner to Vitamin C

Vitamin E was discovered at the University of California in Berkley by Dr. Herbert Evans in 1922. Since then, it has become well accepted as nature's most effective oil (fat/lipid) soluble antioxidant. It plays a crucial role in protecting cell membranes from oxidative free radical damage. Adequate use of Vitamin E, both internally and externally, can provide protection to oil/lipid cells from the increasingly high free-radical concentrations caused by air pollutants and a lifestyle that exposes the body to oxidation and radiation.

Vitamin E, helpful in the formation of red blood cells, is found in:

- Nuts
- Vegetable Oil
- Wheat Germ
- Leafy Green Vegetables
- Seeds
- Olives
- Asparagus

Most doctors recommend more supplements (200 IU to 800 IU) than can be reasonably consumed in foods. Externally applied supplements have been found to be a significant benefit to skin; however, clinical studies have determined that at least 5% of a solution must be Vitamin E to receive those significant benefits.

In the skin, Vitamin E is found in significant amounts in the lipid compounds in the thin sheets of the stratum corneum, the uppermost surface layer of the skin. Because most of the water cells are located beneath this layer, this is one important reason the use of Vitamin E is so imperative following the application of topical Vitamin C. The application of 5% Vitamin E can help drive the Vitamin C into and through the upper stratum corneum sheets and other layers of the skin to reach the abundant reservoirs of water cells below. This creates a trans-epidermal seal to hold in moisture.

Natural Vitamin E vs. Synthetic Vitamin E

Research indicates that the body cannot often distinguish between natural and synthetic vitamins. Vitamin E is an exception since there are chemical differences between the natural and synthetic forms of Vitamin E.

Roche has been the most reliable and probably the largest supplier of Vitamin E to companies worldwide in the past two decades. According to their reference guide, "d-alpha-Tocopherol" (natural Vitamin E) has a greater biological activity than dl-alpha –Tocopheryl acetate (synthetic form of Vitamin E) on a weight-to-weight comparison.

Besides tocopherols – which include four forms of Vitamin E (d-alpha, beta, gamma and delta), there are other four forms of Vitamin E called tocotrienols, of which there has been less research and fewer findings. Research at the University of California at Berkley suggests that alpha-tocopherol is by far the predominant form of Vitamin E in the body. If you are looking at labels on skin care products, you might have a difficult time distinguishing between the natural and the synthetic form. The new International Nomenclature of Cosmetic Ingredients (INCI) standard for product labels standardizes all Vitamin E as "tocopherol," thereby leaving the question open as to whether the vitamin is natural or synthetic.

Products that use the natural form usually indicate this on the front or back label. Still, if you are unsure, you can call or write the manufacturer and request documentation indicating the form of Vitamin E used. Again, natural Vitamin E is the d-alpha tocopherol form and synthetic Vitamin E is usually dl-alpha tocopherol, also referred to as tocopherol acetate.

Studies in the past decade have demonstrated that natural Vitamin E is not only better absorbed than the synthetic form, but also better retained in the body. This suggests that for external use, natural Vitamin E would also absorb faster through the skin and be retained longer in the skin cells. However, synthetic Vitamin E is still very valuable since most studies have been done using this form. And it was the synthetic form that was used to determine the minimum of 5% to provide the clinically proven benefits. Therefore, this suggests that 5% of natural Vitamin E is more than is clinically found to be needed to achieve benefits.

Effective Application of Externally Applied Vitamin E

The use of this important vitamin applied to the skin at least twice a day aids in the protection of the upper layers of the skin. However, it is important that you know the amount and form of the vitamin that you are applying. To assure you are receiving the maximum benefits, the following standards are recommended:

1) Minimum Percentage – Using only a small amount of Vitamin E on your skin has little performance benefits. The minimum percentage of Vitamin E in a formula should be 5%. Studies using formulas with less than 5% have not demonstrated to have the significant ability to improve the structure of skin. However, the use of less than 5% might have some value as an antioxidant protector.

2) Natural Form – Again, the natural form of Vitamin E has been demonstrated to absorb faster and be retained longer. Synthetic forms of Vitamin E are beneficial, but if you want superior results, natural Vitamin E is the most effective form.

3) Stable to Remain Active - Vitamin E is much more stable than Vitamin C. Still, Vitamin E will lose its effectiveness if it is stored in a warm or hot area for a long period of time. It is important to store your Vitamin E personal care products in an area that is not in direct sun and is relatively cool to assure its maximum efficacy.

Benefits of Vitamin E

1) Provides antioxidant protection
2) Protects against UV radiation
3) Improves elasticity and firmness of skin
4) Acts as a trans-epidermal seal
5) Softens and smoothes skin
6) Inhibits and reduces scar tissue

1) Provides Antioxidant Protection - Vitamin E scavenges free radicals in oil cells just as Vitamin C does in water cells. The ability for Vitamin E to donate an electron to an oxidative free radical that has just lost an electron can immediately normalize the cell again so that it is not damaged and does not continue to damage other surrounding cells.

2) Protects Against UV Radiation – Vitamin E is not a sunscreen as the FDA recognizes sunscreens. However, it is a highly effective scavenger of free radicals that can form in oil cells and therefore can protect the skin from some damage caused by the sun and oxidizers.

3) Improves Elasticity and Firmness of Skin – Malonyldialdehyde (MDA) is a waste by-product of lipid peroxidation, which is part of the cross-linking of collagen. When MDA is created from oxidation of collagen, the result is a loss of elasticity of skin, increasing wrinkles, and breaking down the fiber of the skin, characteristics of aging skin. MDA levels appear to be less when Vitamin E has been used, suggesting that Vitamin E can help slow this process of collagen breaking down.

4) Acts as a Trans-Epidermal Seal - Vitamin E has the ability to help keep moisture in the skin while allowing important nutrients out through the sweat. The ability to prevent trans-epidermal water loss is one of the most important characteristics of Vitamin E in the role of helping prevent the signs of aging.

5) Softens and Smooths Skin – Vitamin E's ability to hydrate the skin helps to improve the feel of the skin. Since it is compatible with the lipids that surround and hold together the surface keratin proteins of the skin, Vitamin E offers great benefits to the health and texture of the skin cells.

6) Inhibits and Reduces Scar Tissue – Probably the most common use of Vitamin E has been in the healing process, since it has demonstrated the ability to help slow the formation of scars, affecting the otherwise abnormal synthesis of collagen that can form a scar.

Vitamin E is a powerful antioxidant by itself, but becomes even more beneficial when paired with Vitamin C.

Vitamin E & Vitamin C are Better Together

The only thing better than using the L-ascorbic form of Vitamin C and the 5% natural form of Vitamin E separately is using them together. Vitamin C appears to travel deeper and is more concentrated through the lipid layers of skin if it is used in conjunction with Vitamin E, especially natural Vitamin E. Vitamin E appears to have more activity when used in conjunction with Vitamin C. It is as if the Vitamin E gains more antioxidant power when it is used in conjunction with the L-ascorbic acid form of Vitamin C, both when ingested internally and applied externally on to the skin.

There are significant amounts of research that demonstrate these vitamins together are more effective. Just as some of the early research from the 1970's led to my interest in the external application of vitamins, more recent research is confirming our claims of the past two decades that applying both Vitamin E and Vitamin C along with a sunscreen is much more protective for the skin and hair than the use of a sunscreen alone or used with either of the vitamins separately.

As a researcher, formulator and educator of product technologies, I have been very conservative in our claims. However, since we have been responsible for the application of over 60,000 pounds of vitamins to human skin over the past ten years alone, we have discovered natural solutions to many conditions of the skin that are sometimes considered diseases.

We do not claim to cure these diseases; however, we can testify that tens of thousands of people have experienced significant benefits to their skin, scalp and hair as a result of being "In the Mode" with the two step application of 12% L-ascorbic acid form of Vitamin C followed by the application of 5% Vitamin E.

We have discovered that Vitamin E and Vitamin C when used together can help normalize the appearance of the following conditions:

- Acne
- Age Spots, Keratosis & Comedones
- Broken Capillaries
- Burns
- Chemically Peeled Skin
- Cradle Cap
- Contact Dermatitis
- Dandruff – Itchy, Flaky Scalp
- Diaper Rash
- Dry, Irritated Hands

- Eczema
- Poison Ivy
- Psoriasis
- Reconstructive Surgery
- Rosacea
- Skin Cancer & Skin Growths
- Sunburn
- Swimmers' Oxidation
- Wounds
- Wrinkles, Fine Lines & Signs of Aging

Other Free Radical Scavengers

Twenty years ago, the FDA was very strict on the claims that could be made about wrinkles and the treatment of signs of aging. By the mid-1990's, companies began making claims that had never been made before, overwhelming the FDA with new and conflicting research that was coming from colleges and companies that were seeing significant changes in the skin by using various ingredients in the lab.

You should understand all of the ingredients you are applying to your skin. You need to know what you are using and what benefits to look for on the label. There is presently information overload in the media, as many companies are making significant claims about slowing the aging process; many different ingredients are being touted as the "latest great miracle."

Following are some of the other ingredient categories—enzymes, minerals and extracts—that also provide skin performance and protection. Still, the safest and most beneficial vitamins for the skin are Vitamin C and Vitamin E—2 two steps in 2 minutes 2 times a day.

Extracts

Extracts are a category of ingredients receiving attention. Grape seed, grapefruit extracts, green tea and pomegranate are some examples of antioxidants that are trends in personal care. There is research that shows these and other extracts, including some essential oils, have antioxidant benefits. As long as these extracts are not intended to radically exfoliate the skin and remove any of the important skin layers, these extracts might have benefits to the skin.

However, if the extracts are fruit acids such as glycolic or other alpha or beta hydroxy acids, you need to be very cautious with their use. The increased usage of these extracts might be the most serious and potentially harmful trend in skin care. My concern about this trend and potentially dangerous lifestyle choice is explained in depth in Chapter 14, which discusses skin exfoliation and treatment services.

Because there is no standard or indication of concentration of acids indicated on labels, the use of fruit acid extracts for radical exfoliation is not recommended. Due to the ease of use and the potential for removal of valuable superficial skin cells, there is little reason to use this approach in skin care when Vitamin C and Vitamin E provide both skin protection and help normalize the exfoliation rate of the skin rather than speed it up.

Enzymes

Enzymes are believed to be even more effective free radical scavengers inside the body than vitamins. Most of the research surrounding enzymes, such as SOD, suggest that the superiority of enzymes over vitamins such as antioxidants taken internally is due to the stability and ability of enzymes to be active even after battling with oxidizing free radicals. Antioxidant vitamins are effective only as long as they are stable and still have any "power left in them."

Antioxidant power comes from their ability to donate an electron, and once the vitamin donates all their available electrons to the previous free radical (to help normalize the free radical to become a healthy molecule), the electrons are used up and the vitamin is not a vitamin any longer.

So, why do we not hear more about enzymes in personal care products? First, because there is still a lack of evidence that externally applied enzymes are superior. Enzymes are difficult to stabilize and synthesize into an effective delivery system to benefit the skin in order to be able to replace or supplement the application of vitamins.

Within the next five years, I expect you will begin to see the use of externally applied enzymes. However, be very wary of any product for skin or hair that touts the benefits of enzymes. At our Malibu Wellness Institute, we suggest that skin and hair professionals, along with their clients, demand from any manufacturer whose products claim benefits from enzymes for documentation of clinical studies of the effectiveness of the enzymes in their product.

A popular antioxidant often categorized as an enzyme is the coenzyme Q-10, or ubiquinone. As a fat-soluble antioxidant, it has been promoted as a contributor to fighting free radicals in the lipid walls of cells. Even though some consider this antioxidant valuable when applied topically, there are questions about the ability of the size of the molecule to be able to penetrate and the ability for the dead proteins in the surface layers to benefit from its presence.

Some enzymes in skin services that dissolve proteins are being used for radical exfoliation. Some of the more popular are papaya enzymes, called papain, and pineapple enzymes called bromelain. The use of these enzymes as radical exfoliation treatments are discouraged and not recommended for Total Oxidation Management, since they are dissolving away the lipids holding the proteins that are important to the protection of the skin. Never consider enzyme treatments that radically exfoliate a lifestyle choice since the short-term benefits are not worth the potential long-term damage.

Minerals

The topical application of mineral compounds, has become another trend in skin care. Having spent almost two decades researching the detrimental affects of minerals such as copper, calcium, and iron on the hair, I find the benefits of most of the products using topically applied minerals questionable. I do not question the need for adequate minerals for internal use, but I am very aware of some of the problems these minerals cause when the skin and hair are exposed to them in excess.

On the other hand, most of the benefits I am aware of that are associated with claims made about the topical application of copper in personal care products can be achieved with the correct use of Vitamin C and Vitamin E, rather than including another step of copper, calcium or any other mineral. Additionally, consumers should question the amount of copper peptides being used in many of the skin care products claiming clinical benefits. Again, minimum percentages should be declared on all skin care products with claims of active ingredients.

Still, the use of minerals such as copper peptide is usually not associated with radical exfoliation; therefore the use of these ingredients is not considered dangerous and there is less caution regarding these ingredients as compared to many of the other popular skin care ingredients that are intended to radically exfoliate the skin.

Of all the minerals, I recommend zinc to be the most important as a topical mineral. Zinc, especially in conjunction with some antioxidants, has been found to be effective in killing bad bacteria that could otherwise cause infection in and on the skin.

Spin Traps

Spin Traps, a.k.a. PBN (Phenyl Butyl Nitrone), might be thought of as the intelligent antioxidant! It is a form of nitrogen, engineered into a unique compound that is proving to be superior in helping normalize free radical molecules, especially internally. Spin traps are claimed to convert free radicals back into vital oxygen to again be effective for respiration of cells, which is necessary for all healthy cells. Research by academic leaders such as David Becker at Florida International University suggests that the use of spin traps has significant potential for both internal and external conditions.

Since spin traps help normalize a free radical to become a stable molecule, I consider this a positive contribution to Total Oxidation Management for the body. To date, however, most of the research on spin traps has been on internal conditions, such as the treatment of blood-flow blockage, stroke, heart attack, Alzheimer's disease, and even hair loss. There is evidence that spin traps might become the first treatment of its kind approved exclusively for strokes, one of the leading causes of death.

Recently, spin traps have become more popular in skin care products. The caution in the use of spin traps is much like the caution of other valuable ingredients – the percentage of the ingredients, the delivery system and the confidence of whether there are enough of the true nitrones to penetrate and be beneficial in the skin cells. And even though one of the benefits of spin traps is the ability to be absorbed by both water and oil cells, the use of spin traps as an exclusive skin care system is not a complete regimen. Still, I am confident the use of spin traps will become a new trend in skin care technology in the next decade.

Chapter 6

T O M

TOTAL OXIDATION MANAGEMENT

Living "In the Mode"
2 Steps...2 Minutes...2 Times a Day

The last chapter explained the many ingredients that are now on the market which claim to provide significant skin care results. Before we discuss how simple skin care should really be, you need to understand the difference between normal and abnormal skin.

What is "Normal" Skin?

You probably define normal skin as skin that looks and feels good, that doesn't itch or hurt, and shows little signs of stress and aging. Total Oxidation Management considers "normal" to be what scientists have discovered is the average condition of healthy skin. What is regarded as "normal" is, in essence, the condition of healthy skin cells from a large sampling of the largest number of healthy subjects, especially younger adults who have less environmental damage to their outer cover.

Reference to "normal" or "normalizing" suggest that with proper attention to the known elements that accelerate skin damage, oxidation/free radicals, we can all slow and perhaps even reverse some of the damage using the correct vitamins in the ideal formulations.

Normal for you is the condition of your healthy skin cells. Look at the inside of your arm or your side...that area might be an indication of what normal skin cells are for you. So the objective of Total Oxidation Management is to prevent oxidation and return your skin to a more normalized condition.

This is a lifestyle change, and the reason Total Oxidation Management is so important. The goal is to achieve and maintain the most normal skin possible by avoiding the conditions that could speed up oxidation. The following signs of aging are categorized as abnormal skin.

"Abnormal" Skin

Abnormal skin is not necessarily diseased skin. So many of the surface skin conditions on millions of people are simply related to the oxidation, past and present, of the environment around them. Some of the most common conditions that appear to be connected to oxidation and an abnormal exfoliation rate include:

- **Dry/Rough/Thick Skin** – Usually caused by the thickening of the outer layer of the skin where the waterproofing ceramide/keratin proteins have been damaged.

- **Fine Lines** – The breakdown of keratin proteins in the outer epidermis layers of the skin.

- **Wrinkles** – The breakdown of collagen in the deeper dermis layer of the skin.

- **Dark Spots** – Often referred to as hyper-pigmentation, spots which occur as the result of hormones, post-peeling procedures, and sun damage. Most often associated with age spots, melanin is pigment or color that accumulates in the skin. As we age, we tend to lose a number of pigment-producing cells, resulting in more pale, translucent skin. The color-containing cells that are left tend to get bigger and group together. This is the primary cause of age spots and they are usually found on skin that has oxidized free radical damage due to exposure to the sun.

- **Light Spots** – Hypo-pigmentation is usually associated with the absence of pigment found on normally dark skin where melanin or pigment has been affected. Some conditions of hypo-pigmentation are genetic; however, these light spots are usually caused by the oxidation of skin and the formation of free radicals that seem to affect an otherwise normal pigment condition.

- **Sagging Skin** – Technically referred to as laxity, due to the loosening of the elastic quality of the skin. Lack of muscle tone under the skin can also contribute to a sagging look to skin.

- **Solar Comedones** – Sometimes referred to as "senile" comedones, these usually become visible on the face, especially the cheeks, in middle-aged and elderly people who have been exposed to sunlight over a long period of time. Affected skin may become yellow and "leathery", at which time it becomes known as solar elastosis or Favre-Racouchot. The comedones may appear as a blackhead which is more open, or a whitehead, which is more closed. However, these comedones are not related to acne vulgaris, the bacteria known to cause acne.

- **Keratosis** – Also known as solar actinic, this condition results in scaly or crusty bumps that form on the skin's surface. The bumps range in size and color and are often detected more by touch instead of sight. They can itch or feel "prickly" especially after exposure to sunlight. This condition is categorized as pre-cancer and can lead to the formation of squamous cell carcinomas. Sun exposure is the cause of almost all actinic keratoses.

Caring for Your Skin

Whether your skin is normal or not, how to care for your specific skin condition can be confusing, since you're bombarded daily with ads about the latest trends in skin care. My concern is that most of the new products on the market are trying to include the most recent ingredient technology combined with extra ingredients designed to speed up exfoliation.

Some skin care companies have as many as 40 different products, with the message that different skin types need as many as six layers of products. I disagree. Skin care should be simple and logical. The goal of superior skin care for every skin type is to provide protection and performance. This goal alone will deliver the fastest benefits with the fewest potential side effects.

With just two steps, Total Oxidation Management is a fundamentally simple approach to skin care, giving you everything you need to prevent the signs of aging and correct some common skin conditions. While other products may be used in conjunction with them, these two steps alone will provide significant results.

Step 1:
12% L-Ascorbic Acid Form of Vitamin C

Throughout this book, we've emphasized the importance of using a 12% solution of the L-Ascorbic Acid form of Vitamin C applied two times a day, morning and night. This first step is the most important element of Total Oxidation Management and is the foundation upon which your entire skin care regimen should be built, since it has immediate lasting benefits.

The combination of the vitamin's performance inside the cells, along with the protection to the outer layers of the skin, make this step necessary for everyone, no matter what your skin type. I am unaware of any other vitamin, mineral, enzyme, extract or engineered technology that is more important, more versatile, with more benefits.

Any Vitamin C serum complex you select should not have the active ingredients (the vitamin) already mixed in with the solution. You or your skin care professional should activate the ingredients prior to your first application to guarantee effectiveness. The most convenient and most logical is to activate the vitamins for one full container that will last approximately one month. Any Vitamin C product that you activate should not be exposed to heat or the sun, so if there is a need for a longer stability, store it in the refrigerator. However, this is not necessary if you keep it out of the sun and if you plan to use it within 30-45 days.

Also, look for a Vitamin C product that is blended with a vegetable gum (e.g. xanthum or cellulose) for even distribution, which assures the quality of the product and allows natural absorption by the surface layers of the skin. Some products are using silicones as a base; however, our research has found most silicones are blocking , counteracting the benefits. Believe it or not, the correct formula using Vitamin C should be so safe it could be eaten, even though that is not the intent nor do companies recommend it. Still, it is nice to know that you are using a product around your lips, your ears and nose that is safe if you happen to ingest some.

More is not better. Just one drop of a Vitamin C serum on the fingertip is enough to cover each section of your face. One application covering your face every morning prepares your skin for the rest of the day. Frequent application might be important if your skin is in an aggressive oxidizing environment or you work outside, but a light to moderate amount is all that is necessary.

This complex is also the one product that can be used to attack skin conditions (see Skin Conditions & Testimonials in the back section of this book) to normalize your skin with no harmful side effects.

Step 2:
5% Natural Vitamin E

The second step to Total Oxidation Management is the use of a moisturizer that includes no less than 5% natural Vitamin E. The benefits of Vitamin E and the advantage of its natural form were explained earlier. However, the need for moisture cannot be over emphasized.

Many women are accustomed to moisturizers that include a complex of various oils and silicones to make the product and the skin "feel" smooth or slick. Slick moisturizers are usually not the ones that would be ideal for Total Oxidation Management, since they likely have too little antioxidant protection and too many ingredients that could be "comedogenic," allowing sebum to build up and block pores, causing acne.

When you think of the word moisture, you think water. However, most moisturizers are not water, but some form of oil. This is because the most important aspect of a superior moisturizer is its ability to create a trans-epidermal seal to keep the water in the cells below and still allow substances to pass through in the sweat to the outer surface of the skin.

Look around and try to find a product that contains 5% Vitamin E, research has found the amount to be the minimum needed to provide benefits. Most companies prefer to include 1% or less because Vitamin E is "tacky" and difficult to break up into small particles for easy application. It took us 13 years before we felt we had created a superior product with all the necessary variables in a 5% hydro-moisturizing formula.

In addition to the importance of the trans-epidermal seal, Vitamin E is an important carrier of Vitamin C—driving it through the oils/lipids down to the water cells below the surface layers. This is the reason we recommend application of the 5% natural Vitamin E moisturizer after the application of the Vitamin C. They not only work more efficiently together, but the Vitamin E helps the Vitamin C absorb through the surface layers into the depths of the skin to reach the dermis. This technology helps stimulate the "factories" that are responsible for the development of collagen in skin.

While all you need to protect your skin, reduce the signs of aging and treat some skin conditions are these 2 steps 2 times a day, other products are explained below that may provide some additional benefits.

Cleansers, Astringents & Scrubs

Cleansers

Cleansers are intended to remove things, not put things on the skin. When you hear the many ingredients that some skin care includes in a cleanser, you have to question how the skin can absorb the ingredients when the most important aspect of a cleanser is to remove dirt, make-up and other impurities that can build-up and block the pores.

Also, if you are using a superior shampoo on your hair and scalp, remember that it is also a great product on your face. Your scalp is also skin, so don't underestimate the ability to cleanse your face in the shower. If you do, it is unnecessary to cleanse your face again.

Still, the time to use 2 steps in 2 minutes is following your cleansing, usually twice a day. Is the right cleanser important? Yes, and it must remove your makeup effectively and leave your skin in a condition that is clean without being dry.

I am making the assumption that cleansing the face is already a part of your daily routine. We have spent years formulating cleansers that provide the correct balance for most skin. Still, the cleanser itself is not the answer to Total Oxidation Management. It is only a precursor.

Additionally, we strongly disagree with skin care companies who recommend Alpha or Beta Hydroxy acids in their cleansers to speed up exfoliation. If you don't know the pH and the percentage of these ingredients, you should not use them at all. Any benefits you can achieve from a pH of around 3 in a concentration less than 30% can probably be better achieved with at least a 10% Vitamin C in a pH of around 3.

Vitamin C has much more benefits with more far reaching results on the skin. The concept of "exfoliating the skin" is too broad and potentially dangerous. However, a system that uses Vitamin C immediately after cleansing normalizes the natural rate of exfoliation rather than speeds it up.

Toners and Astringents

Neither toners nor astringents are recommended as a normal step in Total Oxidation Management. For years, a toner was recommended to women to close the pores, while removing excess detergents and water-element residue from the face following the use of a cleanser.

First, the use of the Vitamin C in a pH of 3 will provide the necessary conditions to help normalize the enlarged pores. This is often seen as early as 28 days from the day the Vitamin C is first used on the face; sometimes sooner, although sometimes it takes months to see significant changes in your complexion.

Second, the surfactants (bubbles that lower surface tension on skin) being used in most facial cleansers are not the same harsh ingredients used years ago when there was residue left on the skin. Therefore, we do not recommend even needing a toner, and this is an unnecessary step if you are using a Total Oxidation Management approach to skin care.

An astringent, on the other hand, tightens the skin and is a product that might be very beneficial to skin that is prone to excessive oily conditions and/or the presence of bacteria, as is often found in acne prone skin. Still, an astringent must be formulated with ingredients that will kill bacteria and remove excess oil. Therefore, use it at the end of the day to remove the bacteria, but avoid overusing an astringent, since it can remove important oils that help seal in moisture in lower layers of the skin. Overuse of an astringent can also dry the skin, leading to additional problems.

Mud Masks

Products that include mud are used to extract sebum and other substances, such as dirt in the pores. Since they are usually a higher pH and are not a radical exfoliant, using a mud mask is very compatible with Total Oxidation Management, although not one of the daily steps.

Used mostly on normal to oily skin, most mud masks are designed to clear the pores, tighten the face, remove dead cells from the skin and leave a smooth texture to the skin surface. Most often, mud is applied wet and allowed to remain on the face ten to thirty minutes. At least ten minutes is usually necessary for most mud compounds begin to dry and leave the smoother feel following application. Once the mud is removed with water and possibly a wet cloth, skin is usually left feeling better than before the application.

Be aware that since mud masks are designed to remove build-up from pores, it could be followed by isolated acne as a result of not fully extracting the sebum. Usually a mud mask would not be recommended for sensitive skin conditions, such as rosacea, until the skin is normalized. An application of a freshly activated Vitamin C in a pH of around 3 would normalize the skin and minimize the irritation and inflammation around the affected area.

Usually, not every mud or clay mask is right for every skin type. Various forms of clay and mud masks are very effective, but some might cause irritation to the skin. Avoid mud products that contain AHA's or BHA's, especially if the pH and percentages are not on the label. Since mud or clay products are often in a high pH to open the pore, AHA's or BHA's that are used in a pH or percentage that is inappropriate for your skin could cause irritations and serious problems. You don't need these additional ingredients, and you certainly do not want to speed up exfoliation during a mud extraction.

Skin Scrubs

Scrubs are most often associated with compounds containing some ingredient that agitates the surface layers of skin to normalize the exfoliation rate designed by nature. Usually these scrubs should be used by applying with the palms of the hands to assure there is not an aggressive contact with the skin. If the scrub states it is for exfoliation, just understand it should help normalize, not speed up, exfoliation below the superficial layers of the skin.

Avoid any scrub that includes the use of AHA or BHA acids. By combining a physical exfoliant with alpha or beta hydroxyl acids, a product could speed up exfoliation, and that is not a Total Oxidation Management approach to skin care.

As you can see, caring for your skin with a Total Oxidation Management approach is a logical regimen to protect against factors in your environment that are causing you to age, which you will learn about in the next chapter.

- The L-ascrobic acid form of Vitamin C in a pH of 3 might tingle or sting slightly for a few seconds. I tingle every morning when I get "In the Mode" on that part of my face where I shave. Stinging indicates you have cellular tissue exposed and not well protected by the stratum corneum layer of the skin   If it stings for a few seconds, give it a few days and the stratum corneum surface layer will likely be normalized and the skin will no longer tingle or sting upon application, unless you shave that area and you are constantly removing that surface layer exposing it to the environment.

- A moisturizer is responsible to create a trans-epidermal seal in the skin holding in moisture while still allowing other cellular functions. Vitamin E is the best natural approach to creating this seal, but it need to be in a solution of no less than 5% to be versatile in its benefits to the skin.

- Vitamin C and Vitamin E products that contain no fragrance will be less likely to cause irritation. However, if you do not like the smell of fresh vitamins, you might want to consider enhancing the product with an essential oil.

- Store your Vitamin E & C in a cool, dark place like in the bathroom cabinet. Both Vitamins E & C hate sunlight. Sunlight or just heat alone will begin to cause both vitamins to loose some of their potency.

- If you have an oversupply of either Vitamin E and especially activated Vitamin C, store the product in the refrigerator and it might stay effective for years.

- If you are using cortisone and possibly prednisone on your skin, the benefits of Vitamin C might be compromised.

- After you have been "In the Mode" covered with Vitamin C & Vitamin E for 28 days, if you stop using the products your skin will likely revert back to its original condition prior to using the 2 steps in 2 minutes 2 times a day.

Chapter 7

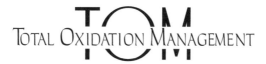

TOTAL OXIDATION MANAGEMENT

The Air Quality in Your Environment Ages You

Oxidation and free radicals surround you, aging the very fabric of your skin. But you can manage how slowly or how quickly it occurs with Total Oxidation Management.

The challenge is to visualize ahead. What might look good or feel good today might be what ages and even destroys you tomorrow. Remember, oxidation and free radicals are slow acting, so the results might not show up for years to come.

Once you understand what oxidizes your skin, you have the ability to decide for yourself how much oxidation you want to expose yourself to–and that's where Total Oxidation Management begins.

Oxygen + Environment = Oxidation!

Only a few extra ingredients combined with oxygen are necessary to accelerate oxidation to the point that it can lead to damage. When oxygen is combined with the sun, water and/or chemicals, liquids, and gases, the oxidative processes that wear down surfaces, such as metals, fabrics and skin, begin. If oxidation can fade your blue jeans or a flag flying in the breeze, just think how it can tear down your skin's cellular tissues.

Air Pollution Speeds Up Oxidation

Do you hear any reports or discussion about the pollution in your community? It might not even be coming directly from your neighborhood, but blowing in from surrounding areas. The air pollution surrounding you refers to gases that contaminate pure, and otherwise, natural conditions. This contamination by pollution creates free radicals in the air, on your car, and on your hair and skin.

Air pollution affects humans internally in three ways:

1) Pollution particles or gases are absorbed through the skin.

2) Gases or small pollution particles are breathed in.

3) Pollution particles are eaten in food or water.

Pollution Inside: Home & Work

The air in your home is probably more polluted than the air outside your home! The American College of Allergists suggests that half of all illnesses are either caused by, or made worse by, indoor air. Much of the problem stems from our desire to be energy efficient. By tightly closing our houses and workplaces, we have created an environment where pollutants are unable to escape. Additionally, many of us have higher levels of pesticides and other pollutants inside our homes than are found outside.

A cigarette is the indoor pollutant that causes the highest amount of oxidative free radicals to the largest number of people. The trillions of free radicals that can form from a burning cigarette can affect everyone in the environment. Smoking in a home or car with innocent developing children should be illegal, since the effect on children can last forever.

Many people spend over a fourth of their life in the workplace, causing more and more states to become aware of pollution that can exist at work. This is evident in the number of cities and states that are banning all smoking from public places and adhering to the guidelines provided by the Environmental Protection Agency.

However, the air pollution elements in many businesses are not always as obvious as cigarette smoke or the fumes from dry-cleaning and printing odors, but rather something as simple as a heating or cooling unit that emits polluted gases. This is one reason proper ventilation is so important in the work place.

The greatest damage results from the combination of many elements combined together to cause a polluted environment. For example, salon professionals make most of their money oxidizing hair in an oxidizing environment! Studies suggest that the incidence of asthma among salon professionals is higher than that of the general population. Additionally, the numbers of salon professionals who smoke cigarettes have greater chances of developing long-term damage to both their internal and external body.

For example, it's not unusual for professional stylists to have dry, irritated hands, which are the result of rinsing hair saturated in chemicals used to oxidize—or bleach and color—hair. Not only are stylists also regularly exposed to oxidizing chemicals such as bleach, perms and straighteners, the air itself is full of chemicals, making Total Oxidation Management especially important to hair and nail salon professionals and their clients.

Pollution Outside: Air & Water

Research suggests that in developed and rapidly industrializing countries, the major outdoor air pollution problem is most often associated with high levels of smoke and sulfur dioxide. This form of air pollution comes from the combustion of sulfur-containing fossil fuels, such as coal for domestic and industrial purposes. Sulfur dioxide gas reacts with oxygen and atmospheric moisture to produce conditions such as acid rain and smog.

However, the major threat to air is traffic emissions. Petrol and diesel engine motor vehicles discharge a variety of pollutants, specifically carbon monoxide (CO), oxides of nitrogen (NOx), volatile organic compounds (VOCs) and particulates (PM10). Photo chemicals react with sunlight to accelerate the oxidative processes that produce free radicals, resulting from the action of nitrogen dioxide (NO2) and VOCs from vehicles. This in turn leads to the formation of ozone, a secondary long-range pollutant that travels to other regions of the country far from the original site of emission.

One result of the many emissions of pollutants is how the moisture in the air also becomes polluted, which can lead to acid rain. It's clear how acid rain affects plant life, but most people do not understand what it can do to their hair, skin and scalp. Acid rain can cause itchy skin, hair loss, and salon service failure.

Once the air quality is compromised and the formation of water from that polluted air begins to fall, the water passes through the layers of earth known as "aquifers." These aquifers are most often layers of rock.

The more acid the pH of the water, the more the water tends to break the rocks into smaller and more concentrated particles. The water now has a much higher content of dissolved solids than it otherwise would have contained.

This water is then pumped, usually through metal pipes, creating even more minerals in the water, which is then used in homes or businesses. This is one reason we find that water has a higher concentration of dissolved solids and metals, which increases oxidation and contributes to common problems such as dry, itchy skin and conditions such as eczema and psoriasis.

The next chapter describes in more detail what may be hiding in your water that affects your hair and skin.

Chapter 8

TOM
Total Oxidation Management

The Water in Your Environment Ages You

Once you understand what's hiding in your water, you may spend less time relaxing in a warm shower or bath. Elements in the water that affect your skin may not be obvious; however dry, itchy skin or dandruff, eczema and psoriasis may be linked more to your water than to a medical condition.

We have found many skin conditions of children that are caused by what is in the family's water. You will read in the Skin Conditions & Testimonials how Total Oxidation Management has changed the lives of families whose children suffered from severe skin conditions that were compounded by the water in which they bathe.

The likelihood is high that the water you use every day could be contributing to some of your skin conditions and signs of aging. Three types of chlorine compounds are usually added to water:

1) Chlorine Gas

2) Calcium Hypochlorite Tablets

3) Sodium Hypochlorite Solution

I have been testing chlorine and mineral content in water around the country for two decades, and the concentrations of both—especially lime or calcium—have as much as doubled in some communities! The following explains how both chlorine and minerals can affect the skin.

Chlorine is All Around You

When the element chlorine (a high-energy salt) is added to water, it combines with the oxygen in the water to produce an aggressive oxidation reaction intended to kill pathogenic bacteria and viruses. Chlorine's "cousin" chloramines are a combination of chlorine and ammonia and are not as good at killing bacteria as chlorine, but are often found in water that has a higher pH. Water that contains chlorine or chloramine can affect the skin.

You know what chlorine bleach can do to your clothes. The fading and weakening effect on fabric is a good example of what an oxidizer can do to the fabric of your skin and hair. Just as chlorine lifts pigment to lighten fabric, it also wears or ages the fabric by oxidation.

Total Oxidation Management might be more important to swimmers than to any other group of athletes, since they are faced with constant exposure to chlorine and minerals, which together accelerate oxidation and destroy skin and hair cells. Once swimmers understand how the water in the pool affects their skin, they can adjust their lifestyle to combat the constant oxidation.

Since chlorinated water is an oxidizer, exposure increases the free radicals that form in otherwise healthy skin cells. When chlorinated water evaporates on the skin, even more damage can occur. If there is any exposure to sunlight either while in a pool or outside a pool, the oxidation process is even more accelerated.

Minerals are Invisible Rocks!

What's good for the inside of your body is not necessarily good for the outside of your body. You may have read about the importance of taking calcium and other minerals internally. These minerals are good for your hair and skin when they are ingested. They do not travel to the outside of the body like vitamins. However, when minerals are in water and exposed to your hair and skin, they can create abnormal conditions for your skin and scalp.

Minerals that adversely affect skin and hair (remember, there is hair on your skin)

- Calcium (lime)
- Iron
- Copper
- Magnesium
- Lead

What is Hard Water?

It is important to remember that some of the best water for drinking might be the worst water for the healthy condition of your skin and scalp skin. If you have hard water, you might also have:

- Dry, flaky or itchy skin.
- Symptoms much like that of dandruff, eczema, and psoriasis of the skin and scalp skin.

77

The presence of calcium (Ca) and/or magnesium (Mg) in water categorizes water as being "hard." Calcium is either found naturally from the ground or added to the water by the treatment plant. More than 70% of the water pumped into homes in the U.S. is hard water, and over 60% of water pumped into homes in Great Britain is hard water.

The American Society of Agricultural Engineers has classified water hardness as:

- **Soft:**   0 –60 parts per million
- **Moderately Hard:** 60 – 120 parts per million
- **Hard:** 120 – 180 per million
- **Very Hard:** more than 180 parts per million

Hard water does not necessarily contain other minerals, but people often think of iron when they think of hard water. And yes, iron can be contained in hard water, but it is not always present. Calcium and/or magnesium are always present in hard water. Unfortunately, you cannot easily see calcium or magnesium in the water as it flows from your shower, but you can see or feel the effects.

You Could Have Hard Water If:

- Lime-scale deposits form around the sink and basin.
- It is difficult to create a lather.
- It is irritating to dry skin and infant skin.
- You have eczema.
- Blonde hair darkens or hair color fades after two weeks.
- You have hair loss.

A Closer Look at What Comprises Hard Water

Calcium (Lime) - Calcium can be found in both surface water and ground water. Calcium is found in limestone, and is also in the lime that is added to water during the treatment

78

process. Lime is Calcium Hydroxide or Ca (OH) 2, a positively charged mineral. The addition of lime to water acts as a binder of elements and can raise the pH of water (often necessary because the alum that is added during the treatment process is an acidic salt that lowers the pH).

The calcium component in lime can have a negative impact on the hair and skin. The calcium is invisible and attaches on to the hair like a magnet, contributing to conditions such as hair loss or flaking on the scalp skin, often thought to be dandruff. Salon services that "fail" (such as hair color, straightening or perming) is usually the direct result of calcium oxidizing on the hair and creating a wall that blocks the chemicals from processing properly. This will be addressed further in an upcoming book.

Magnesium - Magnesium is often found wherever calcium comes naturally from the ground. It's abundant in the soil and is very much a part of the mineral complex associated with hard water.

Iron - Iron is found in ground water from domestic wells, ground water used by treatment plants, and is also often found in water that is transported through old iron pipes in older communities.

Copper - Three different sources for copper in water include:

- It comes from underground and is pumped into the water from a well.

- Particles of copper can come from copper piping. The corrosion caused by chlorine and other elements can cause scaling and lift copper particles off the pipes and deposit them into the water.

- Copper sulfates are added to swimming pools to control the growth of algae. This is also occurring in many reservoirs that use copper to control the algae during the warmer months.

Lead - According to the EPA, lead can be found in homes that were built prior to the 1950's. That includes many wonderful cities (including New York, Boston and Toronto, as well as many other "old towns") with lead pipes, and homes that were built between 1982 until 1987, when copper pipe with lead-based solder was banned from use on domestic drinking water plumbing. Copper pipes are still used today, but lead is no longer being used as the basic solder material. It was found to be "not such a good idea," and the elements from the lead were removed in future homes. Still, many people are drinking and shampooing in water that might not be very healthy.

Lead acetate is also used in certain home remedies for gray hair cover-ups. Lead darkens the hair. It also causes serious problems if an oxidizer such as peroxide is applied over it.

Hard Water & Skin

Scientists in Nottingham, UK reported a study conducted at the Queen's Medical Centre at the city's University Hospital., whereby more than 4,000 local primary school children were found to have more cases of atopic eczema in the areas where residents were showering with hard water.

The study did not conclude the exact cause of skin conditions due to exposure to calcium, magnesium, and other minerals in the water, but the study certainly confirms our experiences and why we feel that our 2 steps in 2 minutes 2 times a day, along with vitamin bath crystals, can help normalize skin conditions.

The pH of Your Water

The "p" stands for "potential" and the "H" stands for the element "Hydrogen." So, pH is the "potential for Hydrogen." Therefore, pH is the amount of free hydrogen ions in a water solution. Simply put, pH is a measurement of water (sometimes referred to as an aqueous solution). Oil does not have a pH, wood does not have a pH, hair and skin do not have a pH—only the water solutions that are most closely associated with your skin and hair have a pH. Sweat from your internal body and the water you shower with, plus the products you put on your skin, constantly affect the condition of your skin.

The pH of your internal body is a measure of your bodily fluids, such as blood, intestinal excretions, urine, saliva, and sweat. Most research is pointing to the need of maintaining a pH of around 7, which is a neutral pH. Research suggests that a diet heavy in protein and even most fruits causes an "acidic" condition in the body. If your body is highly acidic (low pH) and is producing ammonia to offset that condition, the ammonia will be excreted through your sweat glands and can cause abnormal and frustrating conditions as a result of the high alkaline state of your skin and hair.

pH is a very hot topic among medical and wellness experts, with a whole new category of books being written about how a person's diet affects their internal pH. A trend in nutritional circles is the use of coral calcium and pH buffers to help manage internal pH. This new trend is making a difference in many conditions that were otherwise misunderstood—it is important to realize that your internal pH does affect your external pH. Still, diet is both the problem and the solution.

You have heard about "pH balanced" soaps and shampoos. You need to understand what pH balance means uniquely for you since the specific water you use affects your skin and hair. There are varied views of the best pH for hair, but usually around 5.5 is considered most common. However, the shampoo and soap that you use are only on your body for a very short time. For many people, the pH of their water might affect them more than the pH of the soap and shampoo. The pH of all three is important. Water is the first and last thing on your body when you bathe. And, as previously mentioned, many water companies add lime (calcium) to the water to raise the pH so that there is less corrosion to the pipes.

The pH of your water is important, and a good reason to use Total Oxidation Management during and following bathing to maintain the health of your skin. If you understand what pH is, you can immediately change some of the conditions of your hair and skin while managing your oxidation.

How Does a High, Alkaline pH Affect Skin?

Skin appears to exfoliate more normally and experience less abnormal conditions when it is in an acidic environment. A condition of a high pH usually would occur as a result of either a diet that produces ammonia coming to the surface of the skin through sweat or from the pH of the water and/or products used on the skin. Probably the worst condition of skin would be exposure to hard, chlorinated water with a high alkaline pH – and there are many community water systems that have just these conditions. You can look at your annual water report to help you determine if your water has some or all of these conditions.

Our 2 steps in 2 minutes 2 times a day after every time you cleanse with any type of water can help immediately normalize the skin, returning it to a more optimal acidic condition and free of oxidizers.

Measuring pH

You can determine the measurement of pH in your water, and even in your saliva, by a simple litmus paper. Even though it is not the most scientific measure, it has proven to be an indicator in chemistry classes for years. The simplest explanation of pH is the measure of whether something is more acid or more alkaline. And the more extreme a solution is—acid or alkaline—the stronger and more aggressive the pH has on people and things. Take a couple of minutes to study the following diagram to help you better understand pH:

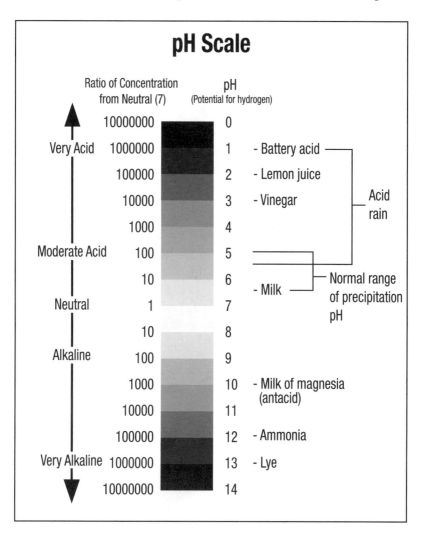

The chart above demonstrates the significance of the differences in pH. It would be logical to assume that if 7 is neutral, then the difference between 7 and 8 is half as concentrated as the difference between 7 and 9. However, as you can see by the chart, the pH of 8 is *10 times* more alkaline than neutral (7) and the pH of 9 is *100 times* more alkaline than neutral (7). When we understand that the pH used in chemical peels is between 2.5 and 2.0 which is respectively *50,000 to 100,000*

times more acid than what is found at neutral (7), it is no wonder a chemical "acid" peel dissolves the protective surface layers of skin right off your face.

Any extreme acid or extreme alkaline is caustic and has serious affects on most substances. As you begin to understand the significance of pH, what the pH of your water is at home, what the pH is of the personal care products you use, along with the services you allow on your body, the more motivated you will become to live a life of Total Oxidation Management.

Now that you understand how the water that surrounds you is affecting your skin, let's examine how these elements can be oxidized even more by the sun.

How to Test Your Water:

- **Chlorine** - Purchase a chlorine test kit from a pool supply store. This kit should include Orthotolidine. The cost is usually less than $10. (Note: dry test strips are not as reliable as orthotolidine to indicate chlorine). When you are ready to test your water in your shower or bath, turn the cool on and allow it to run for at least one minute. Fill the vial with water as instructed on the kit directions and add drops of orthotolidine to indicate the level of chlorine. Testing your water at different times of the year will often indicate different levels of chlorine. Usually, higher levels of chlorine are found in the summer and fall due to higher levels of bacteria found in water during those times of the year. The higher the level of chlorine, the more potential for affects of oxidation on your skin.

- **Minerals** - The most common minerals found in water that can affect your skin and hair are calcium and magnesium. The levels of these minerals can be easily tested with a hardness test strip. Levels exceeding 120 parts per million are considered hard and over 180 parts per million is excessively hard. Hard water combined with chlorine can accelerate the oxidation of the minerals and compound on your skin and hair. The easiest way to indicate your hardness level is to review your annual water report or call your water company for a copy of your report. You can also receive a test strip by visiting www.WellnessSalon.com and clicking on "Ask a Wellness Advisor."

- **pH** - You can purchase a simple litmus paper to indicate whether your water is acid, neutral or alkaline. You can purchase this test at a pool supply store for less than $10. Even though there is some indication litmus paper is not a reliable, it will give you some idea of the pH. The fastest way to determine the pH of your water is to review your annual water report provided by your water company. The ideal pH for water on skin would be neutral or slightly acid. However, most water systems are indicating higher levels of pH rather than lower levels as they do not want the acid to deteriorate the pipes underground. Our research has indicated there are water companies with a pH as high as 10, which is very alkaline.

Chapter

TOTAL OXIDATION MANAGEMENT

The Sun in Your
Environment Ages You

Sun is possibly the leading cause of oxidative free radicals, and it certainly appears to be the major cause of free radical damage to skin tissue. Rather than being an oxidizer itself, the sun's radiation is a catalyst for the process of oxidation that converts a perfectly healthy molecule in your skin cells to a damaged, free radical molecule.

Sun damage to the skin is progressive and accumulates over time. The skin has a memory, and years of exposure to the sun, tanning beds and even reflective UV rays from pool water, sand, and snow can cause progressive free radical damage to the skin. The American Cancer Society predicts over 51,000 new cases of skin cancer each year, so it's time for everyone at every age to take notice of how the sun can cause damage, especially skin care professionals.

Part of the reason for increased cases of skin cancer may be that the ozone layer is getting thinner, allowing more ultraviolet rays to reach the earth. Fair-skinned people who have the least protective melanin are the most susceptible. But even those with dark skin can develop many signs of aging caused by the sun if there is a lack of Total Oxidation Management.

Sun is Energy!

Sun is a good thing; for example, it helps us produce Vitamin D. However, much like oxygen, too much of a good thing can be bad for you. To understand why, following is an explanation of the sun's effect on skin.

The sun is made up of various intensities of energy. This energy involves electricity, magnets and radiation, appropriately called "electromagnetic radiation." This energy travels in waves to our earth. Just as a wave of the ocean has high and low points, so does the sun's energy, such as light, has crests and valleys. The distance between the top of each crest is the wavelength, and the number of ups and downs per second is the frequency.

Imagine holding one end of a rope while the other end is tied to a door knob. When you vigorously move the rope up and down, it creates crests and valleys. You know that the faster you go, the more ups and downs and the smaller the crests and valleys. That means that the faster the frequency (number of ups and downs) of light energy, the smaller the wavelength (length between the waves).

So what does that have to do with you and your skin? We seem to be directly affected by only a narrow spectrum of the energy that the sun generates. What we see, what contributes to our food sources, and what causes damage to our skin is mostly from ultra-violet (UV) energy wavelengths.

UV Rays

Ultra violet rays and infrared rays each interact with the oxygen on earth in different ways. Infrared light has a longer wavelength than oxygen; therefore, the "red wavelengths" pass the oxygen without interacting. However, the blue or ultra violet wavelengths are very similar to the wavelength pattern of oxygen. Look at it as if the wavelengths are two ropes about the same length that being shaken up and down at about the same speed.

Since ultra-violet rays are "riding a similar wave" as oxygen molecules, the oxygen atoms cause the violet or blue light to scatter. When they interact together and scatter, the blue bounces off the oxygen molecules.

This is why the sky appears blue violet and also the reason the sky is the bluest in the middle of the day when there is the greatest amount of light energy. This is also why the bluest sky is found where there are few pollutants that cause free radicals affecting the oxygen molecules. Excessive exposure to this ultra-violet light energy bouncing off the oxygen molecules increases oxidation.

When there are pollution particles in the air, there is more oxidation. If you live in this type of environment you are oxidizing faster.

Ultra-violet light is measured in nanometers (nm) on a scale of 100 to 400. The rays that directly affect our skin measure between 280-400, even though some research is indicating above 400 might still be affecting our skin. The following chart might help you better visualize these measures:

UV Ray	Spectrum 400nm down to 100 nm.	Effect on skin
A (UV-A)	400-315	Most past research suggests UV-A rays cause skin to tan and not burn. However, recent research reports that UV-A rays can also cause free radicals and damage the t-UA molecule that can lead to fine lines and even might be a catalyst for cancer.
B (UV-B)	315-280	UV-B rays affect the skin all the way down to the dermis, the deeper layer of skin where the collagen proteins can be impacted and cause wrinkles. UV-B causes skin to burn and seriously damages deeper layers.
C (UV-C)	280-200	The good news is the UV-C rays do not hit the earth. However if they were able to get to the earth, this spectrum of energy would be very dangerous to skin and life itself as it is absorbed by proteins and can damage the RNA and DNA that can lead to cell mutations, disease and death. Scientists are watching more carefully to determine if UVC rays are reaching the earth.
V (V-UV)	100-200	The Vacuum ultraviolet range is absorbed by almost all substances including water and air, and therefore does not affect skin.

Suntan vs. Sunburn

It has been recognized for years that UV-A radiation causes the skin to tan while UV-B rays cause the skin to burn. This implies a simple assumption that UV-B is bad and UV-A is good; in fact, good enough for UV-A tanning beds to become a viable industry, even approved by the FDA.

In past decades, most research concluded that cancer caused from sun exposure is due to UV-B rays and not UV-A rays. And because it was thought that UV-A rays only penetrate the epidermis and not as deep as the dermis, most experts have taught that UV-A rays could not burn the skin and cause cancer. However, for many years the FDA received numerous comments concerning claims that UV-A rays were, in fact causing damage to the skin. The FDA considered the evidence strong enough to "implicate UV-A radiation as a major cause of, among other things, photo-aging of the skin."

How Do Ultra-Violet Rays Create a Sunburn?

UV-B rays reach the dermis, the lower section of skin where they affect the collagen and can even affect the "factories," the fibroblasts in the dermis layer. Previously healthy molecules that made up healthy protein cells in the skin are "zapped" by the UV-B rays, causing an electron to be released, unleashing a once stable atom that begins "terrorizing" the molecules around it until cells and DNA are affected, thus causing mutations.

Therefore, a sunburn is the result of free radicals being formed. This is why the skin gets red, inflamed, and why a sunburn hurts more the second day than the first. The free radicals are spreading and attacking healthy cells. If the free radicals are able to continue to attack, skin can be radically destroyed.

What's a Suntan?

A suntan is the increase in melanin pigment that causes skin to be darker than normal. A suntan is actually a primary defense in the skin. When the body is subjected to UV-B or UV-A rays, the melanocytes produce more pigment to help prevent sun rays from penetrating the epidermis. The darker you are naturally, the more melanin you can produce, and therefore the more defenses your body provides.

Tanning Beds, Lamps & Salons

Tanning beds fit into the same category as smoking when it comes to Total Oxidation Management. First, tanning beds accelerate the oxidation of the skin, similar to the effects of the sun's radiation, an oxidative practice that creates unhealthy molecules from healthy ones.

UV rays in a tanning bulb are UV-A rays, not UV-B. And since UV-B rays are most often associated with the free radical damage to skin cells, the conclusion of many is that tanning beds are safe.

However, UV-A rays can cause the trans-urocanic acid (t-UA) molecules in the stratum corneum layer of the skin to fold upon themselves and create free radicals that can lead to the aging of the skin and conditions that may lead to cancer.

Tanning Beds + Natural Sunlight = Double Trouble

Many people use tanning beds to prepare their skin for a trip to the beach. My observations are that most people who use indoor tanning beds during the winter months are the same people who enjoy sunbathing during the warmer months.

Research has found that the combination of the two might be even worse than either one alone. Use of indoor tanning bulbs may alter skin cells and actually increase the sun's UV-B's ability to promote the development of skin cancer. Therefore, if you are interested in indoor tanning, it is imperative you understand the implications for the potential of free radical damage that can result from combining indoor tanning with natural sunlight. This is why Total Oxidation Management is so important for your skin — it can be the difference between life and death.

Medications Can Create Photo-Toxic & Photo-Sensitive Allergic Reactions

Medication in a person's system may react with UV exposure to create adverse affects that manifest mostly in or on the skin. The reactions usually occur hours or even days after the initial exposure to the UV radiation.

Photo-toxic chemicals appear to make the skin super sensitive to UV rays, usually causing it to appear similar to a sunburn with extreme blistering and change in skin color peaking within 12-24 hours after exposure. Photo-allergic reactions appear to have a more serious affect on the body and can affect the immune system.

Protecting Your Skin from Sun Damage

Studies in the last five years have caused a shift in opinions that has led to many changes in how we should protect our skin from the harmful effects of the sun. Any ingredient now approved by the FDA for sun protection must absorb, reflect or scatter sun light energy in the ultraviolet range at UV-A, or UV-B wavelengths of 290 to 400 nanometers.

The two most commonly used ingredients now approved by the FDA for UV-A protection are zinc oxide and titanium dioxide. Both of these ingredients provide a barrier that is considered thick enough to prevent the damage that might be caused by UV rays.

Just remember that the best idea is not to tan in a tanning bed and to limit your exposure outdoors. If you do continue to tan, get "In the Mode" with freshly activated Vitamin C followed by natural Vitamin E.

You'll learn more ways to protect yourself from the sun's damaging exposure in the next chapter.

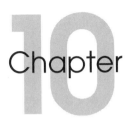

Chapter

TOM
TOTAL OXIDATION MANAGEMENT

All Sunscreens are Not Created Equal

New research has changed the way biologists, chemists, and formulators, as well as the FDA, view UV-A rays' effect on skin. The new findings led to some surprising changes in sunscreen protection. As you learned in the previous chapter, it was once thought that at the higher end of the UV-A spectrum, around 400, there was little or no impact on skin. And that made sense considering that the other end of the spectrum, closer to the dangerous UV-B rays, is where the damage to the skin has most often been observed.

New concerns about UV-A exposure center on one type of molecule in the skin. We have a photo-absorber pigment-like molecule in the top layer of our epidermis—the stratum corneum of our skin—which is called a trans-urocanic acid (t-UA). You'll see all of the layers of skin and their functions in Chapter 11. t-UA was once thought to act like a sunscreen against UV rays.

However, in 1998, two researchers at the University of California, San Diego—Dr. John Simons and Dr. Kerry Hanson—discovered that this molecule might actually be a link to many of the signs of aging caused by exposure to UV-A rays in sunlight. It is interesting that this molecule that was once thought to be "nature's sunscreen" has turned out, instead, to be another target cell where free radicals can produce and lead to changes in skin.

While the t-UA molecule is the "great defender," the two researchers assert that in its attempt to defend, t-UA can go through stages of collapsing upon itself, creating free radicals in the surface layers (stratum corneum) of your skin. These free radicals lead to both an increase in the appearance of aging, and also to specific forms of skin cancer.

These important findings have changed the way the world now views UV-A rays. Prior to their findings, the FDA only required sunscreen ingredients to protect against the UV-B rays. Years ago, PABA (para-amino benzoic acid) was the primary sunscreen that was approved by the FDA for the protection of UV-B's effect on the skin. PABA, as well as most of the sun barrier ingredients approved by the FDA, is effective for the UV-B rays that are most often associated with sunburn free radical formation.

Over the years, many people found they were allergic to PABA, and PABA-free sunscreens became very popular. With the change in regulations, the FDA now requires that a product offer a broader spectrum of protection that includes both UV-B and UV-A rays because of the new research on the t-UA molecule found to be damaged by rays in the UV-A light.

The new regulations and requirements for products claiming to provide sun protection has also changed many views about the "once justified" safety of tanning lamps and beds as we discussed in the last chapter.

The FDA Creates Stricter Sunscreen Regulations

Take notice and you will see that sunscreens are changing right in front of your eyes. Congress mandated the FDA issue new regulations for sunburn prevention and treatment in 1997. And the FDA has done an excellent job of listening to researchers, corporations, and consumers to establish new standards and to make the regulations clearer.

All OTC (over the counter) products that claim to protect the skin against sun damage by declaring a SPF fit into the category of drugs. Some of the changes you will likely notice on the shelf include the absence of sunscreens with a specific SPF over 30, a broad-spectrum of protection statements, water and sweat-proofing, plus new warnings and fewer product claims that were once much too broad and not standardized.

Chemical vs. Physical Sunscreens

The argument over whether a sunscreen is natural, organic, chemical or chemical free is misleading consumers and many are making the wrong assumptions.

ALL sunscreens contain chemicals. The marketing hype of chemical vs. chemical free focuses more on how the ingredients react with UV radiation. Most of the sunscreens use chemical activity to absorb, and therefore, screen, the UV-B rays. Only zinc oxide and titanium oxide scatter or reflect radiation and are therefore considered more of a physical activity. But in reality, both are chemicals in that any two atoms joined together produce a chemical.

Rebecca Gadberry, an instructor of cosmetic sciences, teaches that any compound that joins two atoms together creates a chemical, suggesting the ingredients in any sunscreen formula are chemicals.

Where much of the confusion exists is the clarification of whether an ingredient uses a chemical process or a physical process for protection. For example, Octyl Methoxycinnamate (Octinoxate), one of the most commonly used sunscreen ingredients, is an organic compound that works by absorbing UV-B radiation. Octinoxate uses chemical processes to lower UV radiation energy levels and then releases the energy as heat.

Zinc oxide and titanium dioxide are commonly used sunscreen ingredients used mostly for the management of UV-A rays. Zinc oxide acts differently from Octyl Methoxycinnamate in that it helps physically change the UV-A radiation by scattering or reflecting the energy rays.

SPF Can Be a False Security

SPF is an abbreviation for "Sun Protection Factor." SPF is a well-accepted measure for a product that absorbs UV-B radiation that otherwise causes sunburn or technically, erythema, a skin reaction including abnormal redness and inflammation of the skin. The SPF factor is a measure of how long you can remain in the sun's UV-B rays and not burn as compared to how long you can remain in the sun with no SPF factor and not burn.

I believe it is more logical and technically correct for sunscreens to be identified by their percentage of block (e.q. 97%) rather than an SPF number. No SPF product can guarantee all protection from all UV radiation. In fact, most people assume that if a product has an SPF of 30, you receive double the protection compared to a product with an SPF of 15. Contrary to that assumption, an SPF factor of 30 is only 5% more effective in blocking UV-B rays than an SPF of 15.

The percentage of protection from UV-B rays that can damage the skin:

SPF 15: 92% of protection from UV-B rays

SPF 30: 97%

SPF 45: 97.5%

You can see from this information that the difference in an SPF of 30 and 45 is only 0.5 %. And yet it sounds so...high! The problem is that in the case of a 30 compared to a 15, the benefits are only 5% greater and yet the amount of ingredients used to increase that screen is as high as 300%.

The ingredients that are approved for sunscreens have their down side. Many people are allergic to the ingredients, and many researchers claim that some of the very ingredients that help block the free radicals caused by the sun actually cause free radicals on the skin.

More SPF is Not Necessarily Better

There has been a numbers game going on in the commercial sunscreen business, but the FDA wants to put a stop to that. The FDA, researchers and most doctors agree that an SPF 15 is adequate for most conditions and for the majority of skin. However, some dermatologists and many manufacturers have the opinion "more is better" and have petitioned the FDA to allow the higher numbers.

These high amounts of SPF-approved ingredients have become more for marketing and commercialism and less for the necessity of protection. Therefore, as a compromise, the FDA was considering mandating that sunscreen products exceeding SPF 30 be labeled with SPF values no higher than "30+" or "30 plus."

But, just as this new regulation was to go into affect at the end of 2002, opposition from the medical community and many manufacturers has resulted in a delay on this provision from the FDA. Most of my sources suggest that within two years, the FDA will likely prohibit any SPF of 30 or more to be sold over the counter and instead require these be sold by prescription only.

Don't be fooled into thinking that more is better, and that a higher SPF will provide you absolute protection from the sun. If you plan to be outside with your skin exposed to direct sunlight, you should include an SPF of 15 as part of your protection; and don't be surprised if you still hear many skin care professionals advise consumers that the higher the number, the better. This is, I suspect, more about marketing and the assumption that more is always better, rather than science.

Water & Sweat Resistance Claims on Sunscreens

The FDA has approved a very strict test for a product to claim any resistance to water and sweat. Such a product must retain its stated SPF factor after 40 minutes of being in the water or doing an activity that causes sweat for the same amount of time to be labeled as water-resistant. If the product retains its SPF factor 80 minutes after any of the above, it can be identified on the label as "very water resistant."

A product that is not labeled as water resistant may indeed be even though it is not promoted on the label, since manufacturers have to pay for the testing to have the claim verified. If the label declares "water-resistant," then the manufacturer has paid for the verification required by the FDA.

Still, it is very important to understand that it is difficult for even a water-resistant product to remain on the skin once in the water. Any rubbing of clothes or towels, or sitting in a chair, or even rubbing up against a float or the sand can and probably will remove the protection. Total Oxidation Management includes the practice of re-applying any protection when exposed to the sun for an extended period of time.

Should Sunscreens be Used on Every Body All the Time?

I recently heard an expert on skin care suggest that children from the age of two years should be wearing an SPF 15 at all times. I appreciate the concern that many skin care specialists have for protection, but the sun is also a very important source of positive energy for us. Additionally, with the concerns of some of the approved ingredients in sunscreens,

I am a firm believer that the use of a SPF-approved sunscreen at all times is not only unnecessary, but also not healthy.

Sunless Tanning Products

As you've discovered, tanning using any form of UV rays can lead to damage of the skin. Yet, in the past few years, advances in formulations of self-tanning products have led to new products. The active ingredient that is approved for a bronzing tan without UV exposure is known as DHA. DHA is dihydroxyacetone, which is actually a derivative of sugar. The effect is much like the results of cooking sugar—it caramelizes into a rich dark color.

Research has also found that this use of sugar in the form of DHA might also provide mild protection from the real UV rays. I have heard some ingredient specialists who are confident the proper percentage of DHA applied regularly may provide as much as an SPF 15.

Still, this information has not been substantiated by the FDA; therefore, you will not see an SPF rating on a sunless tanning product unless it also contains approved ingredients included on the FDA monograph for sun protection. Most research suggests that the percentage of DHA in a product to provide adequate sun protection should be 5-6.5% and the product should be applied to the skin no less than every three days.

One downside to DHA on older skin with pigment age spots is that DHA may make the spots much darker.

Adding Vitamins E & C to Sun Protection

For almost two decades, I have been trying to educate professional skin care specialists about the importance of using the ideal form and percentage of Vitamin C and Vitamin E under a sunscreen that includes a minimum SPF 15 for maximum protection.

In the April 2001 issue of *Global Cosmetics Industry* magazine, a report called "Breakthrough in Sun Protection" cited a study that concluded that Vitamin C and Vitamin E "are needed in addition to UV-A and UV-B filters in order to obtain optimal skin protection from UV-induced free radical damage." The study was led by Dr. Kerry Hanson, Ph.D., University of Illinois, who is the same researcher who helped identify the t-UA molecule while he was at the University of San Diego.

I believe very strongly that everyone's skin should be covered with the active L-ascorbic acid form of Vitamin C at every age and all the time. Nature attempts to provide us this coverage, but in this time of extreme exposure to UV rays and the fact that our diets usually do not contain enough Vitamin C to assure that any vitamin makes it to the outer skin surface, it is important to supplement with external application.

This lifestyle change can make a significant difference in preventing free radicals from forming on your skin and help normalize conditions that otherwise could be considered skin irritations. To be effective, use 10% to 12% fresh dried Vitamin C with a pH between 3-3.3, which is a moderate acid as opposed to a radical acid. Additionally, a 5% solution of natural Vitamin E will boost your free radical protection for the oil/fat/lipid cells in your protective skin layers.

Therefore, surround yourself with the vitamins, but be cautious of constantly surrounding yourself with sunscreen ingredients. A good rule is to apply your sunscreen when you know you are going to be in direct sunlight in the mid-day for over thirty minutes, but apply your vitamins every time you cleanse your face and body.

The sun is actually good for us, and we need some exposure to it, just as oxygen is good for us, but not too much to create oxidative free radicals. The Total Oxidation Management approach is moderation, understanding your skin type, and the application of vitamins to protect the layers of your skin, which are explained in the next chapter.

Chapter

TOM
TOTAL OXIDATION MANAGEMENT

Skin is Simple to Understand

Nature is amazing. The way our skin is designed to perform and protect is an engineering marvel and a perfect example of Total Oxidation Management. As you'll discover, understanding how the skin is structured and why it is structured that way is easy—once you understand it, you will be empowered to minimize your signs of aging while preventing how fast future signs of aging might appear.

The most important thing to take away from this chapter is how vital it is for you to protect the outer layers of your skin, since the outer layers are designed by nature to form a barrier against outside intruders.

The method that nature uses to continuously create and protect skin is as beautiful as any story in biology, which we'll go into more detail on the following pages. Simply, baby proteins are born—usually referred to as "daughter" cells—for the sole purpose of being sacrificed to protect us. Once these babies are born, they push up towards the surface of the body every day until they become brick-like barriers cemented together by oil/lipids to create a great wall of protection. Along the way up, these live, plump baby proteins die and change their shape into flat, dead shells of matter that have a specific purpose of protecting our bodies from the harsh world in which we live.

Radically exfoliating these layers, which will be discussed in depth in Chapter 14, is one of the most harmful things you can do to your skin, because it interferes with nature's creation and exfoliation.

To further understand why this outermost layer should remain protected, following is a more in depth explanation of how the components of the skin work together.

The Components of Skin

Skin has defined divisions with distinct layers that include various components, each providing numerous Total Oxidation Management functions. All of these various components together create a substance we call "skin," a flexible mesh of fibers in a complex netting-like matrix made up mostly of:

1) Water cells

2) Protein cells

3) Oil cells

4) Pigment producing melanin cells

The chart below depicts how much of the skin is made up of what substance:

Type of cell	Approximate percentage of skin
Water cells	70%
Protein cells	24%
Fats/Oil/Lipid cells	3%
Other cells including Melanin, Langerhans, & blood vessels	3%

The combination of these cells sits on top of a subcutaneous layer of fats and muscles. This amazing collection of cells serves as a support system for:

1) Protection from physical cuts, and physical and chemical burns.

2) Providing a barrier to help block the entrance of micro-organisms.

3) Helping screen, alter or absorb UV radiation like that of the sun.

4) Transporting water waste and nutrients to sweat glands.

5) Synthesizing pigment for protective color.

6) Synthesizing Vitamin D.

7) Providing support for blood vessels that carry nutrients and moisture to skin cells.

8) Creating "fertile ground" for optimum hair growth

Let's take a look at each of these types of cells individually for a better understanding of their functions.

Water Cells

Approximately 70% of our skin is made up of water, making it the most abundant element in the skin. The water in your cells, water balance and the nutrients found in those water cells are very important aspects of healthy skin.

The blood flow in the skin, along with sweat, transports nutrients to cells while also helping regulate the heating and cooling of our body's internal system. There are as many as 20 blood vessels and hundreds of sweat glands found in and beneath a square inch of skin, in addition to the numerous water-based cells that are important to slowing our signs of aging.

The proper health of your skin cells can affect how well your blood and sweat perform their important tasks for helping to maintain the intracellular water in the cells, while providing other important functions for the skin. Just as your tears help moisten your eyes and keep them normalized, your sweat helps your skin and the entire body be normalized.

And, just as the transpiration of a plant involves water evaporating to create a cooling action, water also evaporates from the skin to keep you cool. But while sweat appears to be cooling the body, it is also transporting many elements that are necessary for skin cells to function properly.

Water is a carrier for nutrients and waste from inside to the outside of the body. You might not be aware, however, that nature is not just eliminating waste; it is also transporting important "hitchhikers" such as the L-ascorbic acid form of Vitamin C. Since Vitamin C is water soluble, it is carried through and to the skin to help scavenge free radicals that can damage the skin and the internal body—another reason this form of Vitamin C is the single most important vitamin in the protection and performance of skin.

Vitamin C is transported to the outside of the skin depending on these variables:

1) How many fruits, vegetables, and supplements are consumed internally.

2) How many internal free radicals use up much of the available ingested Vitamin C.

Because of the inadequate amounts of fruits and vegetables in most diets, combined with the fact that so many free radicals are raging both inside and outside our bodies, applying the L-ascorbic acid form of Vitamin C externally is imperative.

Protein Cells: The Physical Building Blocks of Skin

Layers of proteins that are fibrous matter comprised of amino acids are the life and substance of skin. The water and oil help in the manufacturing, positioning, and stability of these proteins. Therefore, the health of these proteins is what most of Total Oxidation Management of skin is designed around.

The three primary forms of protein that make up our skin include collagen, elastin and keratin. Protein molecules form a chain of two amino acids that are bonded together in a series to form various shapes for specific functions. The specific number of atoms and their arranged order results in the development of a particular protein, some of which are listed below.

1) **Collagen:** Collagen, found in the dermis, is the fibrous protein found in the white tissue of the dermis. These protein molecules are shaped like rods that are bundled together to provide significant strength. Men, by nature, appear to have more natural collagen in their skin, and as the skin becomes more oxidized—especially from sun exposure—free radicals appear to cause the collagen to become thicker. Together with elastin proteins, collagen provides skin both structure and elasticity.

2) **Elastin:** Elastin, also located in the dermis, is a protein found in yellow elastic connective tissue. Chains of elastin protein molecules form rubber-like fibers that stretch much like a rubber band. As the skin gets older and oxidative damage occurs in even normal conditions, the body produces less elastin. Too much oxidation, especially caused by the sun, can cause skin to thicken as the elastin looses its flexibility and the "rubber bands" become twisted and bind together.

3) **Keratin:** Keratin proteins are what form most of our epidermis. Produced by keratinocytes, these proteins are born for the sole purpose of eventually flattening and dying in order to protect our skin from the outside world.

These proteins are all valuable and necessary components of Total Oxidation Management and they should be protected. Even though keratin proteins are referred to as "dead," which suggests they are unnecessary, nature creates these proteins as a method for protection for the lower layers of the skin and the internal body.

Oil/Fat/Lipid Cells: Protecting the Skin's Surface Layers

Often referred to as lipids or fats, oils play a significant role in the structure of skin. And even though oils make up a relatively low percentage of the skin, this percentage is enough to play an important role in the support, feel and health of skin.

Lipids are very important to the natural Total Oxidation Management of skin, since they hold in place the dead proteins that act as a "brick wall" to guard the skin from the harsh environment. The waxy-like substances produced by these cells help the skin to hold in the important moisture inside and at the same time provide a barrier to harsh liquids from the outside.

Comprised mostly of an oil complex of ceramides, cholesterol, and fatty acids, lipids help provide a waterproofing barrier and water binding functions. Lipids are manufactured in little factories called the keratinocytes, the same place keratin protein is produced. As the lipids are released, they divide in layers and rise to the upper layers much like the proteins.

While the role of fats and lipids might appear less important than water since water is so much more dominant in skin, the oils are very significant. As we discussed in Chapter 5, Vitamin E is one of the most important supplements to nature's own system.

Melanin—The Color of Your "Genes"

Melanin from the melanocytes is formed primarily in the basal layer of the epidermis and can rush to the surface in an emergency when exposed to light energy, namely UV-A and UV-B rays. This is what we call a tan. There are two different types of melanin producing cells in the melanocytes of our skin: eumelanin, a dark black-like pigment, and phaeo-melanin, a reddish, brown-like pigment. Asian skin might contain higher levels of beta-carotene that produce a yellowish pigment which can affect skin color and may help slow the signs of aging. For more information about sun tans and sunburns, refer back to Chapter 9.

These cells that are made up of water, protein, oil and melanin make up the two sections of skin: the lower division (dermis) and the upper division (epidermis).

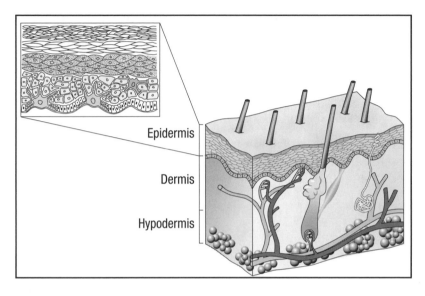

Epidermis

Dermis

Hypodermis

Sections of skin (Figure 1)

Dermis & Epidermis: What Lies Beneath

The Dermis is a Factory

The dermis is like the basement of a building that provides the solid foundation, housing the production and storage of heat and power (collagen protein, blood, and other water cells discussed above).

One of the primary factories in the dermis is known as a "fibroblast," where the key structural components discussed earlier, including collagen and elastin, are produced. The health of the fibroblasts in the dermis section significantly affects the thickness and health of the upper epidermis, the outermost protective cover of your skin.

These fibroblasts also produce and regulate the important cells that lead to the development of the keratinocytes discussed previously. The dermis also serves as the base for hair follicles and roots, nerve endings, sweat and lymph glands.

The two distinct layers of the dermis are the papillary layer and the reticular layer.

a. **The Reticular Layer**—The deepest and largest layer of the dermis. It contains numerous collagen fibers that are bundled together, reaching up into the upper layer of the papillary and also deep into the subcutaneous layer.

These bundles of collagen and elastic fibers lay parallel and are important in the support and connection between the body beneath and the skin upon which it rests.

Below this layer is the subcutaneous layer that is not usually considered part of the skin.

b. **The Papillary Layer**—The smaller layer of the dermis where much of the production occurs. This layer has papillae, or bumps, that lie right on the border of the dermis and epidermis, helping to connect these important sections together.

Located in this layer are connective tissue fibers that contain capillaries and neurons for sensory experience. Blood vessels that pass through this layer carry nutrients and release heat through to the surface layers to cool the body. Additionally in this layer are corpuscles that indicate messages such as touch, pressure and temperature.

It is clear why it is important that there are layers on top of the dermis called the epidermis which protects the dermis from all the intruders that could destroy the body.

The Space Between

In between the dermis and epidermis in the basement membrane are small "spikes" that are protein projectiles of cellular tissue helping to hold the sections together. As oxidation and the aging process continue, these projectiles become less "spiked" and more oval until they are flat-like, which begin affecting the health of the skin cells.

Epidermis: The Defense Department for the Dermis

The epidermis contains four layers (and another additional layer found on hands, feet, elbows, known as the stratum lucidum) and acts as a protector of the dermis. The epidermis is where the oil/lipids, along with the building blocks (keratin protein), color pigment (melanin), and other defensive cells of the skin are located. The four primary layers are:

- Stratum Corneum
- Stratum Granulosum
- Stratum Spinosum
- Basal Section

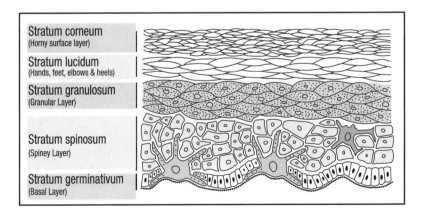

Layers of skin (Figure 2)

Each layer has its own contribution to Total Oxidation Management. You'll see how important the epidermis is in aiding skin's natural ability to manage oxidation and prevent free radicals from destroying the cells that form your skin.

The Life & Death Cycle of the Epidermis

Leaves of a tree grow from the end of the branch toward the sun. In contrast, skin grows from the bottom layer (like the roots) up to the surface. The following is a simplistic view of the mitosis cycle of skin from birth to death until it eventually falls from the body.

Phase 1: New building blocks (keratinocyte proteins) are produced in the basal layer from nutrients and substances derived from the lower dermis section.

Phase 2: Keratinocyte proteins push up the previously made building blocks (keratin proteins) into the spiney layer where the proteins begin to "die" and the remaining cells create a hard shell of lasting protection.

Phase 3: As the keratin proteins die, they continue to be pushed up from underneath, and in the granular layer they begin to flatten out (think of them like a brick) and become surrounded with a wax-like substance (lipids).

Phase 4: Once positioned much like brick and mortar, the dead keratin protein cells take their place as a wall made up of thin sheets in the stratum corneum of the skin, acting as layers of defense. These thin sheets are stacked compactly into approximately twenty-five mini-layers deep. This top layer provides the outer shell for covering and protecting the deeper layers of skin as well as the entire body from environmental elements and UV rays.

The following description of each section will give you a basic understanding of the incredible process of how protein is made, how it dies, and how it is then stacked to protect intruders from entering the skin.

Mitosis
Proteins' Life & Death Cycle to Create Skin Layers

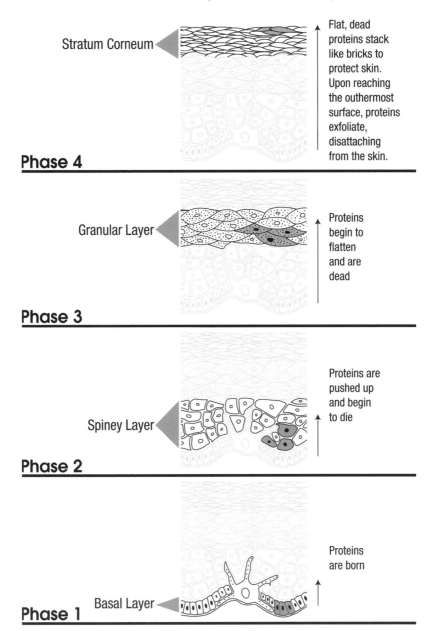

Stratum Corneum

Flat, dead proteins stack like bricks to protect skin. Upon reaching the outhermost surface, proteins exfoliate, disattaching from the skin.

Phase 4

Granular Layer

Proteins begin to flatten and are dead

Phase 3

Proteins are pushed up and begin to die

Spiney Layer

Phase 2

Proteins are born

Basal Layer

Phase 1

Basal Section

The Foundation for Manufacturing Protective Keratin

The deepest layer of the epidermis is the basal (stratum germinativum) layer. This is the base layer where germination of growth comes together and forms the foundation on which the surface layers of skin built. And just as the dermis is characterized as the factory where components are made, the basal layer is more like the center of operations where assembly occurs and distribution begins.

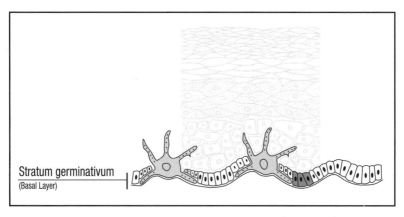

Stratum germinativum layer of skin (Figure 3)

This one single layer of cube or column shaped basal cells form the keratinocytes, where protein is produced. Many of these basal cells are stem cells that constantly divide, allowing one cell to remain as a support cell in the basal layer and the other begins the journey upwards into the surface layers of the skin.

The keratinocytes are cells that are derived from the blood, and include protein filaments called tonofilaments, which contain the necessary ingredients to produce the new fibrous keratin proteins. As new cells are produced, they push up previously developed cells to provide layers of protection until they eventually reach the outermost layer (stratum corneum) and then fall off or exfoliate.

The basal layer allows for creation of numerous other processes and actions that are similar to the environment a seed needs to germinate in the earth. This is unique in that this one single layer is also where the synthesis of our skin color, melanin, has its beginnings. This is where the melanocytes are found, which as discussed earlier are an important part of natural Total Oxidation Management since they protect the skin cells from excess radiation from the sun.

This is the reason a person of African descent has more melanin than a person of Scandinavian descent since the sun exposure to the skin is very different in those respective climates. This also explains why more melanoma, a malignant cancer that forms in the melanocytes, occurs more frequently in fair skinned people than dark skinned people. It is interesting to point out that the number of melanocytes does not vary so much among people. However, the amount of melanin produced in those melanocytes is what separates a dark skinned person from a fair skinned person.

Additionally, the basal section is where Langerhans or mast cells appear to be generated. Even though they can and will travel to upper sections, they are most prevalent in the basal level, where they provide the most activity. The Langerhans cells are another natural form of Total Oxidation Management. They help in the defense against abnormal protein formations and provide an immune response to help "sick cells." Unfortunately, the Langerhans cells are very sensitive to UV radiation and when these cells are destroyed, significantly more unhealthy cells are allowed to form in the skin, causing abnormalities that might be seen in the structure of the skin on the surface.

Additionally, the basal layer is where Merkel cells are found. These cells are especially important for indicating the sense of touch. When pressure is applied, as occurs with touch, these cells compress chemicals that indicate to nerve endings that those cells have experienced various degrees of pressure, and that message is transmitted to the central nervous system.

Protection of the basal cells and all components of the basal layer is imperative to healthy cell development. The need to maintain the surface layers of protection above this basal layer is paramount in the health of the skin. If excess oxidation occurs and free radicals are formed to replace healthy basal cells, a change in the DNA of those cells can result in basal cell carcinoma, a serious form of skin cancer.

Stratum Spinosum: Live Proteins Begin to Die

The layer just on top of the basal layer is the stratum spinosum or more often referred to as the Spiney Layer. This is where the basal cells of keratinocytes in the basal layer are pushed up and where they are tightly bound together by desmosomes. When a cluster of these cells are viewed under a microscope, the desmosomes (that adhere the cells together) appear as spines (such as a porcupine) between each cell. Hence, this is where the name, stratum spinosum, or the spiney layer, is derived.

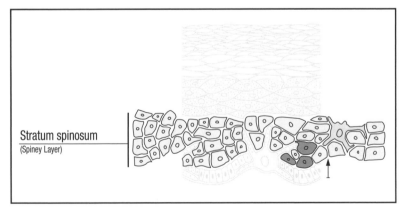

Stratum spinosum
(Spiney Layer)

Stratum spinosum layer of skin (Figure 4)

This thick section of activity consists of 8-10 layers of oval shaped cells fit tightly together. There is an indication that some of the cells closest to the basal layer still divide and reproduce, just as there is also indication that there might be some cells that begin to die in the cells closest to the granular layer just above this spiney layer. You will notice in the diagram on the next page how the shape of the cells begin to flatten out slightly as they are pushed upwards toward the outer layers of the skin.

Also in this spiney layer there is evidence of extensions of both melanocytes and Langerhans that extend to provide defense of the cells in both the spiney layer and the all important basal layer below. This layer is much like a transition layer of protection and synthesis where the keratinocytes change their shape, becoming more oval and begin to die as they move upwards to the next layer.

Stratum Granulosum: Dying Cells Begin to Flatten

As these keratinocyte cells move up from the spiney layer towards the surface, they begin to flatten into granule-like shapes, flatter than the oval they once were, that are known as the granular layer (stratum granulosum). This layer consists of 3-5 layers of keratinocytes that have become much flatter and begin to die. This process begins the formation of what will lead to layers and layers of dead protein that act as bricks in the outermost layer to provide the outermost protection for skin.

This process occurs when the tonofilaments become more defined in the granular layer, while at the same location, a protein called keratohyalin converts the tonofilaments into keratin. These keratohyalin are found in granules that are visible under a microscope, hence the name granular layer. Additionally, other granules in this layer, called lamellar granules, secrete the oil/fat/lipid substance which accumulates between cells and forms the waterproof barrier.

As large amounts of keratin begin to extrude from the cells, the nucleus of the cell degenerates, resulting in the death of the cell. The cell then dehydrates as the remaining cell forms a thick layer of dead matter that flattens out and continues to be pushed up from below. This has created a flatter mass of protein matter that becomes a new, secondary physical layer of protection for the skin layers below. Along with the mildly acidic fluids, fatty lipids, and matter known as ceramides, the cells are tightly sandwiched between the dead matter known as phospholipids.

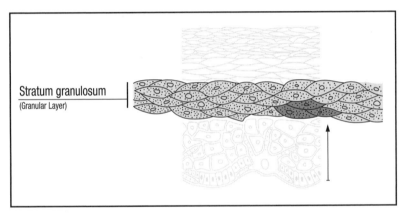

Stratum granulosum skin layer (Figure 5)

It is also in this granular section that the light absorber pigment-like molecule t-UA (trans-urocanic acid) is apparent. At the same time the proteins and membranes degrade, histidine is released, and histidase (histidine ammonia lyase) catalyzes, resulting in t-UA molecules. These important molecules are another form of the skin's natural ability to provide some Total Oxidation Management. These molecules can absorb some of the damaging affects of the UV radiation that could otherwise penetrate to damage the DNA in the basal cells below.

Once this molecule is formed it moves up to the stratum corneum surface area of the skin along with the dead proteins to help provide defense against the sun's UV rays. However, it is important to realize that counting on these molecules for protection is not ultimately a wise idea as they can be damaged by the exposure to UV radiation and eventually lead to signs of aging themselves.

Stratum Lucidum: Hands, Feet, Elbows & Heels

Some skin, such as our hands and feet, require a heavier protection from use and abuse. This additional fifth section (stratum lucidum) lies right between the granular layer of the skin and the thick stratum corneum on the surface of the skin. This additional skin layer is found on the fingertips, palms, soles, elbows and heels where friction occurs to help provide additional defense against invasive wear and tear.

This tough layer of skin is made up of 3-5 layers of clear and flattened dead keratinocytes that are loaded with keratin protein. This additional layer looks clear or transparent under a microscope and appears pinkish to the eye. Still, nature has provided this additional layer for added pressure and physical protection. However, it does not fit so much into the category of Total Oxidation Management, as it is transparent with no melanin.

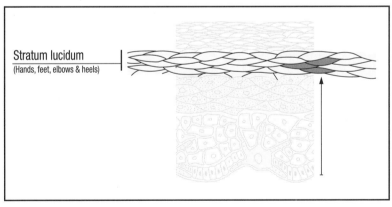

Stratum lucidum
(Hands, feet, elbows & heels)

Stratum lucidum layer of skin (Figure 6)

It could be considered a barrier against oxidizing chemicals; however, we work with hundreds of professionals and consumers who have hands that are affected by the oxidizing chemicals they use in the their work. We know that with the L-ascorbic acid form of Vitamin C in the proper delivery system, the appearance and feel of the hands can be normalized in less than a month and never re-occur.

Stratum Corneum: A Wall of Dead Brick-like Proteins

The stratum corneum (sometimes referred to as the horny layer) is the very top final layer on the surface of your skin that is most subjected to the cruel world outside the body. It is the skin we see and feel every day. It was probably named the horny section because it appears as a tough, protective layer that has an uneven fabric with a weave-like pattern under a microscope. Research on this outer layer of skin suggests that there is more protein (40%), more lipids (20%) and less water (15-20%) than in lower layers of skin.

Just in the past two decades, research has led to a better understanding of the structure and functions of this superficial layer of thin sheets comprised of flat keratinocytes. Inside these dead cells is mostly keratin protein. As the lipid "mortar" that holds them together deteriorates in the outermost sheets, these cells dismantle or slough off (exfoliate), being replaced by cells that rise up from below that began as live proteins in the stratum basal.

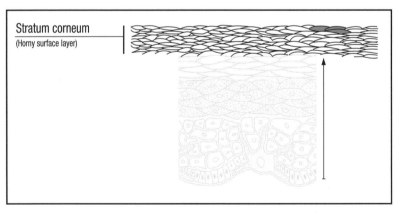

Stratum corneum layer of skin (Figure 7)

Research at Berkeley University by researchers Jens Thiele, Lester Packer, and Maret Traber confirms that this layer is not just a barrier, but actually a "gateway" for transport of particulates, compounds, and nutrients in and out of the body.

Nature has created this top layer, made up mostly of dead keratin protein cells acting as a brick wall surrounded by a waxy-like acid mantle, to provide our first line of defense against the harsh environment we live in.

Some of the protective functions of the stratum corneum layer include:

- Bacterial invasion
- High liquid content (waterproof)
- UV rays
- Physical invasion
- Chemical invasion

There is a constant need to replenish these outermost damaged dead cells and replace them with more recently produced cells that rise up from the deeper layers. However, these proteins enter this surface layer only when they are ready to take on the responsibility of defending the body from the harsh environmental conditions to which we expose our bodies.

The outer layers of skin do a great job of preventing most bacteria, other pathological organisms, and harsh chemicals from causing us harm. Skin was once thought to be a solid armored barrier that nothing could externally penetrate, but is now recognized as a more porous surface area that does allow substance to travel in and out of its mesh-like layers. An example of this is trans-dermal patches, used for nicotine cigarette cessation to transport chemicals directly through the skin and into the bloodstream.

Now that you can visualize how your skin looks and understand the functions of each layer, you can be empowered to manage the oxidation of your skin and slow the signs of aging. You will be able to talk with confidence with your skin care specialist to make your own decisions about your skin.

Remember you should be a partner with your skin care professional in the treatments of your skin; otherwise, you could become a victim of the latest fad and regret that forever. Understand and ask questions.

But most of all, now you are deciding what procedures and daily regimen you choose to maintain youthful, healthy skin. Which procedures are considered to be Total Oxidation Management, and which are not, are explained in the next chapter.

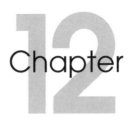

Chapter 12

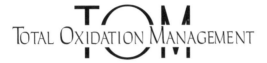

TOTAL OXIDATION MANAGEMENT

Exfoliation

The Second Most Abused Word in Skin Care

Next to the word "antioxidant," the term "exfoliation" is the second most abused word in skin care—and the most dangerous. Consumers and even professionals are led to believe that a product or device is a necessity in order for the skin to exfoliate. This is not true and the confusion is not only misleading but dangerous.

First, let's define natural exfoliation using the simple explanation of skin layers in the last chapter. Nature has designed your skin with a built-in cycle, during which the oldest particles of dead cells on the outermost layer of the stratum corneum fall from your skin and onto your sheets, carpet, furniture, and are even floating through the air.

These particles are actually the "baby" proteins that have risen up through the layers of skin, flattening and dying as they move through each layer with the sole purpose of protecting the outermost skin layers. The flaking off or sloughing off of these now "dead" proteins from the body is the process of "exfoliation." You exfoliate every day of your life.

Normalizing Exfoliation vs. Radical Exfoliation

Normalizing the exfoliation rate helps the very outer layer of skin to slough off at a more normal rate. For example, the use of Vitamin C in a pH of around 3 is just enough activity to help agitate the lipids holding the very outer proteins together and allow those dead proteins to fall gracefully without digging deeper into the protective layers. At the same time, the Vitamin C provides many other benefits, including protecting the skin from the formation of free radicals to promote healthy collagen production down below.

On the other hand, *radical exfoliation* is the use of other acids, such as glycolic, other AHA or BHA ingredients, that dissolve the lipid oils that are holding the dead proteins in their place. Radical exfoliation services include laser peels, chemical peels and microdermabrasion as well as any other physical, chemical or light energy that is intended to remove the surface layers. We will discuss these services in depth in Chapter 14. Radical exfoliation can be done very easily. I often see free exfoliation services offered "in minutes during your lunch hour." It sounds harmless, yet this process is potentially very harmful.

Another term often used for radical exfoliation is *resurfacing*. The idea is to remove the old skin and allow new proteins to take their place. This concept infers that skin is much like hair. You can cut if off and the new hair does not remember the damage the old hair experienced and you start fresh.

This is not the case with skin. Skin has a memory and the factories (fibroblasts) as well as the Langerhan cells, melanocytes, and other important functional cells are affected by radical peels or radical exfoliation. Over several months, some of the same old signs of aging reappear or new ones appear, leaving the client or patient feeling they need to again experience exfoliation or resurfacing.

Yet, when you hear advertising on television and even by many skin care educators about products or devices that claim to "remove dead skin cells to reveal youthful proteins," the message suggests that dead proteins are bad. These messages also infer that removing all these dead proteins will also "stimulate the collagen" in the skin layers below. This all sounds wonderful. Why didn't nature think of it?

Don't Fool Mother Nature

"Remove dead protein cells to reveal new youthful proteins" is like saying "Get rid of all adults, and let the young rule the world." First, the adults might be older, but they are using their experience to make things better for the world tomorrow. The fact is the youth are not ready to rule the world. They still need to grow, mature and experience to be ready to move into that position of responsibility.

The young proteins are not yet ready to be exposed to the harsh environment from which they are expected to protect the skin. This is a serious mistake and a serious misunderstanding on the part of both consumers and some skin professionals. The point is that nature has built in this automatic process of exfoliation. The goal of Total Oxidation Management is to help the skin normalize its natural exfoliation rate rather than speed it up.

Accelerating nature's exfoliation process can leave the surface of the skin very exposed to all the simple oxidizers mentioned previously in this book. Removing even some of those protective layers leaves our skin vulnerable to significant damage that might not show its signs for a few years, but the free radicals that are formed after one single exfoliation service is reason enough to stop and think long and hard before you make the decision to remove the surface layers of the dead proteins.

Radical Exfoliation (Resurfacing) is *NOT* a Lifestyle

Many proponents of radical exfoliation often refer to shaving as an example of why it is a good idea to radically exfoliate as a lifestyle. They will make reference to how the areas where men shave appear to wrinkle slower than the other areas of the face. This argument is a weak attempt to justify the removal of surface protection cells. Where skin is shaved every day is where substantial oil is present and the hair that is immediately growing back provides some of the protection for the skin.

Radical exfoliation or resurfacing should be considered only as a last resort to changing of the physiology the face or body. This procedure comes with cautions and concerns.

And even though sunscreens are recommended after such services, there are serious concerns:

1) Sunscreens themselves are reported to create free radicals in the skin cells and if the surface layers are torn away, the exposure of these SPF ingredients are potentially dangerous themselves especially in the higher SPF numbers as explained in chapter 10.

2) Recently resurfaced skin that is exposed, directly or indirectly, to cigarette smoke is a very serious danger that sunscreens were not intended to (and cannot) prevent.

3) The use of sunscreens can provide false security to someone who has recently experienced a resurfacing procedure and encourage them to go on with their normal routine that might include hiking, swimming, or other lifestyle of oxidation exposure.

Those Who Face the Most Damage

Have you noticed that the individual most seeking radical exfoliation happens to be the fair-skinned woman who is beginning to show signs of aging? There are many statistical reasons why this group will continue to be the victims of these radical exfoliation services.

First, a fair-skinned person had less melanin for protection when they were young. Exposure to oxidizing elements when they were young has most likely led to the formation of advanced signs of aging.

The accumulation of pigment in the form of age spots begins to occur usually after the age of 40. Fair-skinned women in this age group begin seeing signs of aging and feel they are no longer "turning heads." Longing to return to "the way it was," these women decide to have a peel. Very often the woman in her 40's or 50's is the same woman who tanned or burned in her youth. Both tanning and radical exfoliation are short-term benefits that lead to long-term signs of aging.

Second, clients or patients of African or Asian descent have learned that their skin should not be in any way peeled. The amount of pigment is greater in dark skin and the chances for abnormal pigment production following such a procedure are high.

Normalizing Exfoliation is Total Oxidation Management

The use of Total Oxidation Management with 2 steps in 2 minutes 2 times a day is a fundamental approach to normalizing exfoliation, while the short-term benefits of a lifestyle of radical exfoliation do not warrant the long-term effects that might show up as early as months, but most likely in years.

It is a shame when a peel results in the formation of a small pigment spot and then the skin care professional recommends another peel to remove the spot—which was created from the original peel. Over time, the spot can get bigger, and another peel is administered on the belief it will help remove this pigment. This is not a healthy approach to skin care and can lead inadvertently to a lifestyle of radical exfoliation.

The advice of a good skin care professional in treating your skin is recommended. Sorting out the right skin care professional is important. You need to know when you should be consulting a dermatologist, a plastic surgeon, and an esthetician. The different types of skin care professionals can be confusing, and are defined in the next chapter to help you select the right one for you, should you choose to seek their advice.

Chapter 13

TOM
TOTAL OXIDATION MANAGEMENT

Your Skin Care Professional
Doctors & Estheticians

More and more women *and* men are seeking skin care services from professionals, which has led to the growth of more skin care specialists in the medical and salon/spa industries.

Not so long ago, patients only went to their plastic surgeon or dermatologist if there was a problem. After the visit, the surgeon or dermatologist would probably not see the patient again unless there was a need for another treatment.

Today, some of these same physicians are offering regular skin care services, such as the skin resurfacing treatments we discussed in the last chapter. However, as you learned, long-term damage can occur following these types of services, especially if you don't choose the right skin care professional.

Perhaps you already have a good understanding of the numerous categories of skin care specialists. But a review might help to determine who you should be conferring with when you are considering a specific treatment or procedure for your skin.

Plastic Surgeon

A *plastic surgeon* specializes in reducing scarring or disfigurement that has occurred usually as the result of an accident, birth defect, or treatment for diseases.

"Plastic" in the phrase plastic surgery is not intended to infer that plastic is used in the procedures. Instead it is derived from the Greek word "plastikos." This term refers to molding or shaping, which still makes sense since it usually involves the re-shaping of some part of the body.

In the U.S., board certified plastic surgeons are doctors who have completed postgraduate training in one of several specialties: general surgery, otolaryngology, urology, orthopedics, or neurosurgery. Following their postgraduate training, plastic surgeons must have also completed a two- to three-year residency program in plastic surgery in a program approved by the American Board of Plastic Surgery. Following the passing of a comprehensive written examination covering their specialty, the doctor is eligible to practice as a plastic surgeon but still must also successfully complete an oral exam by a panel of peers after a year of practice.

Dermatologist

A *dermatologist* is a doctor who specializes in the physiology and pathology of the skin with an emphasis on the diagnosis and treatment of skin diseases. In order to be a certified dermatologist in the U.S., one must have graduated from a medical school that is identified by the American Board of Dermatology and have a full and unrestricted license to practice medicine or osteopathy in the U.S. or Canada. To be certified, a dermatologist must complete four additional years of postgraduate training as specified by the American Board of Dermatology.

Esthetician

An *esthetician* (also spelled "aesthetician") is a professional trained in the application of beauty treatments such as facials. This relatively new field is licensed by states rather than by a national association and usually is regulated by each state's board of cosmetology.

Being Aware of Your State's Regulations for Estheticians

The requirements for licensing are varied depending upon the state. For example, Alabama requires the most education to become an esthetician—1,500 hours of training and an additional 3,000 hours (approximately 1 year) of apprenticeship to become a Managing Esthetician. Also in Alabama you can choose to take continuing education and become a licensed Master Esthetician. In contrast, Alabama's neighbor to the south, Florida, only requires 260 hours of training with no additional provisions for Managing or Master status. Our research finds that 600 hours is the average number of hours required by states to receive an esthetics license. It is interesting that some states, including Virginia, do not have any license provisions for estheticians.

The scope of services that are offered by estheticians is not consistent from state to state. For example, the state of California allows their licensed estheticians to perform services that include chemical peels to remove the epidermis layer of the skin, which are referred to as "dead layers of skin." Many states have not been so specific; therefore there is still confusion in some states as to what their scope of services allowed within their regulations.

Paul Dykstra and Nancy King are leaders in the cosmetology industry who are working to help regulate the legislative efforts to standardize and protect estheticians and their clients. Together, they have researched and reported information that helps demonstrate the confusion and challenges client/patients have in putting their skin in the hands of licensed estheticians.

The general observation is that newly licensed estheticians are constantly pushing the scope of services that their license legally allows them. In presentations to the industry Dykstra and King report, "The scope of service by an esthetician is to cosmetically enhance the appearance of the skin through non-systemic procedures affecting cosmetics and services, thereby not affecting the cell physiology."

Estheticians & Their Scope of Services

The role of a good esthetician is important; some of the most valuable services they provide are extraction to minimize any over-production or build-up of oil and debris in your pores, as well as screening your entire body to indicate any changes that might be occurring. Those who embrace Total Oxidation Management have a consistent standard, and will help you discover wellness approaches, and can help find areas of your skin that might need medical attention. Additionally, many estheticians offer light massaging of herbs and vitamins (such as C and E) to help provide enhanced results. These services are within the scope of every state's regulations and provide significant benefits.

However, at the same time both the FDA and state departments of cosmetology are becoming very concerned with the number of complaints that are being filed as a result of services that are *beyond* the scope of an esthetician's license. The problem lies in the confusion of what is legally regulated and what is not. For example, many machines that offer services for skin are being sold to salons and spas when in fact the FDA considers them "medical devices" rather than cosmetic.

FD&C defines "cosmetic" to mean "articles intended to be rubbed, poured, sprinkled, or sprayed on, introduced into, or otherwise applied to the human body or any part thereof for cleansing, beautifying, promoting attractiveness, or altering the appearance."

However, it does not include any service that would alter a physical cellular change in skin and certainly not below the outermost stratum corneum layer of the skin. Yet, I am sure you know at least one friend who has been to a salon or spa and come out with a very red, inflamed face. The Federal regulatory agencies are aware of the confusion, but it is presently each individual state's regulatory agencies that are responsible to determine the scope of services of their licensees.

But What if an Esthetician Works in a Doctor's Office?

Rather than the dermatologist or plastic surgeon competing with estheticians, some doctors are *hiring* estheticians. However, it might surprise the doctor, the esthetician and you to know that just because the esthetician is working in the doctor's office, this does not expand the scope of services that can be administered by the esthetician.

In fact, the esthetician might be more limited by what he or she can do than the doctor's assistant, who might have no formal training, because the esthetician is still under the regulations of his/her respective state.

Medical Procedures vs. Cosmetic Beautification

I have some very strong opinions of the important role skin care professionals should and should not play in the care of skin.

For abnormal skin conditions that are causing you pain or other problems, you must determine if a plastic surgeon or dermatologist is right for you. This physician might be the most important person you consult. In this case, you might be seeing your dermatologist or plastic surgeon as often as a few times a year.

However, for beautification to continue to have better looking skin, many people put themselves in the hands of an esthetician every four to six weeks. In this case, your esthetician becomes the biggest influence in your skin care decisions. It is interesting how many people will only visit their dermatologist when their insurance covers the visit; however, that same person will pay cash to their esthetician without thinking twice.

The medical industry is taking notice of the growing number of estheticians who are offering services in salons and spas that are beyond the scope of what the FDA and state regulatory agencies consider legal and safe. This will continue to evolve and consumers will benefit from the safeguards that result.

Choosing the Right Professional for You

The plastic surgeon, dermatologist, or esthetician you choose should first work with you to understand the conditions from which you are seeking relief. If you have an abnormal skin condition, then a treatment might be able to provide solutions without further adverse consequences. However, explore your options and understand the short- and long-term effects of each.

Expect your skin care professional to consult with you to determine the seriousness and urgency of any procedure. Very seldom is a condition on the skin so urgent that it needs to be removed that day.

An urgent removal of any skin condition should only occur if you have determined that an alternative approach using non-invasive approaches, such as a minimum of 10% Vitamin C and 5% natural Vitamin E, did not *normalize* the skin condition. I am still convinced that these two vitamins when used properly can provide solutions to many of the conditions that are afflicting the skin without the many side effects from some prescriptions.

I do not claim these ingredients will cure disease; however, I have witnessed so many skin conditions where the appearance is dramatically improved with these vitamins, that I can only continue to encourage all skin professionals and their clients to give this approach a chance before radical techniques are administered. And if radical techniques are chosen, Total Oxidation Management becomes even more important in the after care as you'll read in Chapter 14.

You can refer to the conditions in the back of this book for in-depth information on wellness approaches to conditions of the skin, including testimonials from people who claim that these 2 steps in 2 minutes 2 times a day have changed their life or the life of a family member.

If you ask them to, some dermatologists and other skin professionals will surgically remove, burn, dissolve or laser the skin right off your face. I once had a dermatologist say to me in response to a keratosis, "What do you want me to do it? I will do whatever you want me to do."

I would like to believe he said that out of respect for my research and position on skin. However, since this dermatologist was unaware of my interest in skin care, I left that encounter with an eye-opening insight that some dermatologists use skin care services strictly as a way to generate income with little regard for the long-term consequences.

I am finding many doctors and skin care professionals who "say" they are not in favor of radical procedures, but they offer them because their clients/patients want them. Just recently, I was told by a spa/salon owner who does not think peels are healthy and "would never have one herself" that she "has to provide peel services that turn the face red (inflammation) or her clients do not think they are receiving any benefits."

Question any skin professional whose first recourse is to dissolve, sand, burn or laser the layers of your face. Generally, I would usually understand the choice of a cutting procedure as done by plastic surgeons to remove layers of skin, since the cut is a specific incision that allows the connective tissues to reform. On the other hand, dissolving or similar techniques used to remove all of an area of skin leaves the entire area much more susceptible to free radicals that can lead to long-term damage.

Still, I have faith in dermatologists and believe that the majority are mostly concerned for their patients' long term well-being. As for my keratosis, it flaked away in less than thirty days with Vitamins E and C: all it took was two steps in two minutes twice a day for twenty-eight days.

If your physician and/or skin care specialist offers you alternatives to peels and other invasive procedures, and helps you determine best regimen with the least harmful short- and long-term side effects, this is the skin professional/partner you want to stay with for life.

The professionals in this group are clearly against radical procedures and don't recommend or administer any chemical or physical peels unless it is absolutely necessary, and then they limit the treatment to the least invasive techniques available.

As new information and procedures become available, do not assume they know more than you. Your research might be more current than their research and, hopefully, they will appreciate your knowledge.

Total Oxidation Management: A Bridge Between Doctors & Salons

The relationship between the medical professional and estheticians has the potential of being a win/win situation for every client. This is the reason we are seeing some doctors align with salons and spas to create a program for clients/patients that is in balance and provides safe and legally regulated services. The adoption of Total Oxidation Management is becoming a common thread that helps these professionals work closely together for the benefit of the client.

Many skin care treatments that are being offered by skin care professionals are described in the next chapter. You are encouraged to research these and other services to best determine if the short term results are worth the potential short and long-term risks.

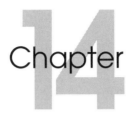

Chapter 14

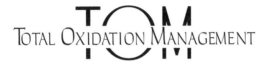

TOTAL OXIDATION MANAGEMENT

Exfoliating Skin Services & Other Treatments

Now that you know what to look for when choosing your skin care professional, you should also be armed with knowledge about different types of skin care procedures.

Radical Exfoliation

We discussed radical exfoliation in Ch. 12, but it bears repeating that radical exfoliation is not a Total Oxidation Management approach to skin care.

A radical peel is the burning, sanding or dissolving away of the wax-like lipids in the surface layers of the skin holding all the dead surface proteins together so that the more recently produced proteins will come to the surface. Removing the top layers of skin theoretically causes a wound-like condition, causing the body to respond by producing more collagen and protein to heal itself.

Radical exfoliation peels are like a burn to the skin. Burns have a severity level, categorized into three types and degrees:

- **First degree burns:** The epidermis layer is affected and removed.

- **Second degree burn:** Skin layers are affected and removed all the way into the dermis layer of the skin.

- **Third degree burn:** Skin layers are affected and removed through the epidermis, dermis and down through the subcutaneous layers of the body.

Because of the damage to the skin, chemical peels have serious consequences, including:

- Increased photo-sensitivity (sun) for up to four to six months following a chemical peel can allow free radicals to form because the skin cells are vulnerable since they are without their mature protective layers.

- Free radical damage can be caused by exposure to direct or indirect sun.

- Any exposure to cigarette smoke (even indirect exposure) for months following a service can cause more damage than the initial damage the treatment was intended for.

- Chlorine and other elements hiding in the water used to cleanse can lead to oxidation that increases free radicals.

- Pollution in the air can lead to formation of free radicals.

- Temporary or permanent pigment lightening or darkening beyond your normal skin color.

- Infection (viral and/or bacterial) can easily take up residence on these exposed raw tissues.

- Scarring can occur over time as this process is an invasive procedure that requires the body to mend itself.

- Contact dermatitis of the affected skin that can be the result of an unknown allergy to medications or ointments ordinarily intended to promote healing. Healing can be prolonged by several weeks with an increased risk of both scarring and long-term skin color changes.

I classify the majority of radical exfoliation services into three categories:

- Chemical (AHA's, BHA's, TCA, and Vitamin A)
- Light energy (laser)
- Physical energy (micro-dermabrasion, sandpaper-like devices)

Chemical Peels & How They Work

The theory of how chemical peels affect the skin is simple. If the surface layers are burned away, much like a wound, the body will rush to repair the damage by producing more proteins. Logic would suggest if you take off the surface skin that is damaged and expose the young protein cells below, the body increases production of more proteins. So how could it be bad? And since the chemically peeled skin might appear more youthful after the healing period because fine lines and age spots have miraculously disappeared, the assumption is that this must be good for you.

Chemical peeling is sometimes referred to as "chemexfoliation." This approach to "radical exfoliation" to the skin involves the application of one or more chemical liquid formulas that use organic acids. Medium peels often contain around 35% acid, although lower percentages can be used for superficial peels to remove most of the epidermis protective layers, and higher percentages (50-60%) are used to produce a deep peel that can reach down into the dermis, removing all the layers of the epidermis and some of the functional layers in the dermis.

These chemical peels are sometimes combined with other treatments such as microdermabrasion, tretinoin cream, solutions of other acids—such as lactic acid and salicylic acid—with the intent of accelerating the results. A procedure is "successful" when the skin care professional has removed all or most of your surface layers of skin.

The depth of a chemical peel is dependent upon the percentage or strength of the chemical and the pH of the formula. The words chosen to describe a chemical peel, as well as other peels, are often misleading. For example, when peels are described as "superficial," one would infer that it is harmless and would have few negative implications. The word "superficial" is ofter used to refer to some or all the layers of the epidermis.

Also confusing is the use of the reference to a "medium depth" chemical peel. This still sounds somewhat harmless; yet, a medium depth peel is usually associated with the destruction of the upper dermis. Destroying all the physical properties and the normal functions of those important layers which might extend down into the factories of the dermis is dangerous and carries with it significant risks. One of the claims often associated with peels suggests that "the deeper the peel, the greater the potential benefits."

But what is often not stated is that this procedure is a more aggressive wounding of the skin with a much longer recovery time and greater risk of complications, not to mention the long-term damage that can occur during the months following when the skin cells are completely unprotected.

Every professional who recommends or uses chemical peels should be completely aware of the concerns that both the U.S. FDA and the European Commission have expressed about the use of such treatments. The following is a statement release from the FDA on December 2, 2002.

"FDA has considered evidence that suggests that topically applied cosmetic products containing alpha hydroxy acids (AHAs) may increase the sensitivity of skin to the sun while the products are used and for up to a week after use is stopped, and that this increased skin sensitivity to the sun may increase the possibility of sunburn. The purpose of this guidance is to educate manufacturers to help ensure that their labeling for AHA-containing cosmetic products is not false or misleading. As an interim skin sensitivity to the sun, FDA is suggesting that the labeling of a cosmetic product that contains an AHA as an ingredient and that is intended for topical application to the skin or mucous membrane bear a statement (of caution)."

Before undergoing a chemical peel, understand how they work,the depth of the peel, why they work, and the many reasons not to use them.

AHA & BHA Chemical Peels

Alpha Hydroxy Acids, and less often Beta Hydroxy Acids, are the most widely used categories of active ingredients used for chemical peels. These "resurfacing" acid facials are provided by skin care professionals. Until the FDA stepped in, they were readily available to consumers in doctors' offices, salons, and even, grocery and drug stores. OTC products with these ingredients are now required to have significantly less AHA or BHA activity, but there is no law requiring percentages be listed on the label.

At our Malibu Wellness Institute, we advocate a standard should be approved by the FDA that pictorially indicates to consumers and professionals the depth of peel range an Alpha or Beta Hydroxy Acid has upon the skin layers. The text or graph should indicate the impact that the percentage combined with the pH within the product will likely have upon the skin layers.

I refer to these acids as radical exfoliants because they can be strong enough to peel away the surface layers of the skin. In order for this to occur, the pH of the product needs to be below 3 and the product must have at least a minimum percentage of the acid ingredient to peel the skin.

Most AHA's are derived from fruit and milk sugars. Sounds reasonable enough. How can that cause any damage? These extracted sugars, however, can create a solution of a low pH acid that can tear through protein layers of skin.

I remember a conversation with an esthetician that stated her number one service was chemical peels. I asked how often her clients returned, and she said she recommend they return every six weeks for another chemical peel service. When I asked if she understood the potential for long term damage, her response was "What else am I going to do to make money?" My response was "Observation, extraction and normalizing services in conjunction with relaxation techniques can bring you much more money with clients returning every six weeks for your services and products."

The U.S. FDA began questioning the effects of these chemical procedures when complaints began pouring in during the mid- 1990's. As AHA's became popular around 1992, it was only a few years later that these complaints led to questions.

AHA's: A List From the FDA

The following is a listing of ingredients recognized by the FDA as alpha hydroxy acids:

- glycolic acid
- actic acid
- malic acid
- citric acid
- glycolic acid + ammonium glycolate
- alpha-hydroxyethanoic acid + ammonium alpha-hydroxyethanoate
- alpha-hydroxyoctanoic acid
- alpha-hydroxycaprylic acid
- hydroxycaprylic acid
- mixed fruit acid
- tri-alpha hydroxy fruit acids
- triple fruit acid
- sugar cane extract

- alpha hydroxy and botanical complex
- L-alpha hydroxy acid
- glycomer in cross linked fatty acids alpha nutrium (three AHAs)

Most often, AHA products sold to consumers over the counter have an AHA concentration of 10 percent or less. The concentration of AHA products used by trained cosmetologists or estheticians may be up to 30 percent, while those used by doctors can range from 50 to 70 percent.

In a report by the FDA, the following was stated:

> FDA has a particular concern about AHAs because, unlike traditional cosmetics, AHAs seem capable of penetrating the skin barrier. In reviewing the limited data on AHAs, FDA concluded in a 1996 report that certain formulations of AHA products can affect the skin in a manner similar to that of chemical peels--that is, increasing cell turnover rate and decreasing the thickness of the outer skin. The effect depends on the product's pH level (a measure of its acidity), the AHA concentration, and the AHA vehicle cream, as well as how the product is used (for example, frequency of use and where on the skin it is applied).

AHA ingredients used in a pH of over 3 and in relatively lower concentrations have little benefit to the skin; however, that is what most of the products on the store shelves include. The marketing of AHA, or more often the popular glycolic acid, is more about the hype than the results. Using these ingredients for their mild acid benefits are insignificant compared to the benefits of using Vitamin C for the same reason. The many other features that Vitamin C can safely provide, makes it superior to AHA and specifically, glycolic acid.

Beta Hydroxy Acids

The most significant difference in AHA and BHA is that AHA is more water-soluble and BHA is more oil or lipid-soluble. As explored in earlier chapters, most of our skin is water, therefore, AHA is going to have more affect than BHA.

AHA is considered to be more effective for thickened, sun damaged skin, whereas BHA is often thought of as more effective for acne and skin that is oily. Still, neither AHA nor BHA acids are recommended as part of a Total Oxidation Management lifestyle for normal skin conditions.

Beta Hydroxy Acids often include the following ingredients:

- salicylic acid* (aspirin is made with salicylic acid)
- salicylate*
- sodium salicylate*
- willow extract *
- beta hydroxybutanoic acid
- tropic acid
- trethocanic acid

* From a chemist's perspective, salicylic acid is not a true BHA. However, cosmetic companies often refer to it as a BHA and, consequently, many consumers think of it as one.

TCA Peels

TCA (Trichloroacetic Acid) is another acid chemical applied only in a physician's office. It is usually slower acting, but still very aggressive and provides a deeper peel than AHA or BHA. The process causes the surface layers to dry and peel away over a period of days to expose the younger, more recently developed proteins deeper in the skin. Often TCA is used for age spots, fine wrinkles and shallow scars.

Phenol Peels

One of the strongest acid peels is a method that uses carbolic acid for deep exfoliation. Called the Phenol Peel, this procedure for the entire face would take an average of a couple of hours, but is rarely used and seldom recommended because of its removal of so many layers of the skin. Such a procedure usually requires mild sedation with a local anesthetic. There are many risks. It takes weeks for new skin to appear and is still pink and sensitive for around two months.

Vitamin A (Retinol)

Vitamin A is vital for helping maintain the structural integrity of cells and the healthy functioning of mucous linings. But a good diet can provide plenty of Vitamin A.

Vitamin A is a fat-soluble vitamin that is found mostly in animal-based foods. However, the body can also make Vitamin A from beta-carotene, a fat-soluble nutrient found in dark green leafy vegetables and the yellow colored fruits and vegetables such as carrots. The liver can store up to a year's supply of Vitamin A. Still, this storage of Vitamin A can be depleted when a person is sick or has an infection.

The external use of Vitamin A is a very complex issue, and just because Vitamin A is included on the label does not assure the user of any of its benefits. Vitamin A is, in fact, very unstable and can cause irritation to many users.

The most common use of stable and effective Vitamin A is by skin care specialists. If your doctor or skin care specialist has recommended or administered a treatment using Vitamin A, read on to better understand how you should be very involved in the decision to have any service using Vitamin A on your skin.

Why Are Dermatologists Recommending A Lifestyle of Vitamin A?

A recent release on the Internet quoted a number of dermatologists who now think that Vitamin A retinoids are the only valuable ingredient in anti-aging skin care. This article published in March, 2003, begins "Cosmetic companies have touted vitamin-based face creams for more than 40 years, but prescription-only treatments containing Vitamin A are still the only scientifically-proven wrinkle fighters, according to dermatologists."

There are plenty of doctors who believe like Dr. Leslie Baumann, professor of dermatology at the University of Miami School of Medicine, who is clearly as passionate about Vitamin A as I am about Vitamin C and Vitamin E. Dr. Baumann was quoted as saying at a meeting of the American Academy of Dermatology, "I highly advise everybody to start retinoids today and stay on them."

I've reached a different conclusion based on years of following research from around the world about vitamins and the skin. In my opinion, the association with Vitamin A applied topically has more to do with the hype of the instant removal of signs of aging rather than the "fighting" of aging. In fact, most of the research shows the folly of that conclusion. The required FDA warnings regarding the use of these ingredients infer that these ingredients may actually lead to faster aging if the user's skin continues to be exposed to sunlight.

Of course, not all dermatologists treat the use of Vitamin A retinoids so lightly; they understand that the use of Vitamin A is not necessarily a lifestyle, but a medical treatment for a specific condition because these treatments are not without risk.

The use of retinoids is serious. If you are using Vitamin A on your skin daily or as a medical procedure periodically, it is imperative that you make the decision on how often you allow these ingredients on your skin, because with the use comes a serious responsibility. And Total Oxidation Management becomes even more important.

Tretinoin: The Active Ingredient of Choice by Many Doctors

Tretinoin—the generic term for Retin-A®—is just one of a number of Vitamin A-derived compounds called retinoids. How tretinoin works is not completely known, but it is well known that the higher the percentage, the more radical the effect on the skin layers. It does appear that there is significant activity which wears through the upper layers of the epidermis, classifying it in my view as a radical exfoliant.

Some History of Tretinoin & Vitamin A in Skin Care Services

Many dermatologists recommend Vitamin A treatments for acne since it has been shown to reduce the production of sebum, which clogs pores. Vitamin A has most commonly been used in a treatment known as RETIN-A MICRO®, using the active ingredient compound Tretinoin, derived from Vitamin A. Tretinoin was manufactured by Ortho Pharmaceutical Corp. of Raritan, N.J., (now owned by Johnson & Johnson, and combined with the Neutrogena Professional division) and has been available by prescription exclusively for acne since 1971.

In 1988, the FDA put out the following statement:

"Retin-A® is approved for use in treating acne. For this use, it is generally applied to small areas of the skin for limited periods of time. Recently, however, the drug received nationwide attention because of a research article suggesting that it may reduce or reverse wrinkling due to aging and sun damage. Reports suggest the FDA does not endorse these study conclusions because of the small number of patients studied and the subjectivity of the observations."

At the same time, Commissioner Frank E. Young, M.D., Ph.D., announced a crackdown on unlicensed manufacturers who have been advertising and distributing bogus Retin-A® drugs.

This has led to Vitamin A treatments being associated with the medical profession as a drug and medical procedure instead of an over the counter cosmetic.

Retin-A® & Anti-Aging

The use of Retin-A® has been approved as a medical service for the treatment of acne. It does not help everyone, but many clients find some relief following a Retin-A® service. However, Retin-A® can cause side effects, the most significant being the decrease in skin pigment and the increase in sun photo-damage that can occur weeks following the service.

I do not recommend Retin-A® as a lifestyle product, and it should be considered only as a treatment for a specific condition. If you do choose this treatment, avoid all direct or indirect exposure to sunlight.

Along the way, doctors began administering Retin-A® treatments for anti-aging purposes. This trend probably began as a result of a report in the Jan. 22, 1988, *Journal of the American Medical Association* conducted by Jonathan S. Weiss, M.D. and colleagues at the University of Michigan Medical Center in Ann Arbor. The study described a 16-week, double-blind study of tretinoin (Retin-A®) cream to treat sun-related skin aging in 30 patients. According to the investigators, all 30 patients showed statistically significant improvements in sun-related skin damage on their forearms and 14 of the 15 patients on their faces.

Even though there might be some signs of aging that were removed from the surface layers, it is important to remember that the outside layers of the skin were removed, exposing the deeper layer proteins that were very young and not ready for the direct sun.

The following is an excerpt from a warning letter published on the Internet to Johnson & Johnson for how they promoted and marketed their product on television. The FDA considers this issue significant enough that they wrote:

"This letter objects to Johnson & Johnson Consumer Companies, Inc. (J&J) dissemination of promotional materials for Retin-A® Micro (tretinoin gel) microsphere, 0.1% that are in violation of the Federal Food, Drug, and Cosmetic Act (Act) and its implementing regulations. Specifically, as part of its routine monitoring program, the Division of Drug Marketing, Advertising, and Communications (DDMAC) has identified a 30-second direct-to-consumer (DTC) television broadcast advertisement (TV Ad) for Retin-A® Micro entitled "Possible" that is misleading. The TV ad fails to clearly communicate and minimizes the risk associated with the use of the product, while simultaneously overstating the efficacy of the product."

This warning also makes reference to and confirms the following warnings that are included with Retin-A® Micro (tretinoin gel) micro sphere, 0.1%: "The most common side effect with Retin-A® Micro is skin irritation. This can include skin redness, burning, stinging, itching, dryness, and peeling. Some of these side effects may go away or bother you less after you have used Retin-A® Micro for a few weeks." It goes on to say what I consider the most important issue, "Spend as little time as possible in the sun. Use a daily sunscreen with a SPF 15 rating or higher, sun protective clothing, and a wide brimmed hat to protect you from sunlight." I recommend the use of Vitamin C and Vitamin E during the day and the Retin-A® at night as a treatment regimen.

More research led to a newer version with less concentration of tretinoin. In the mid-1990's, a new product called Renova® was introduced by Ortho Pharmaceutical and approved by the FDA.

Renova® is Approved For Helping Reduce Skin Damage

The Food and Drug Administration approved the marketing of the prescription product Renova® – 0.05% tretinoin emollient cream – as a treatment to assist in reducing certain kinds of skin damage. The FDA talk paper states clearly "Renova® does not eliminate wrinkles or repair the sun-damaged skin that leads to cancer. Nor is there evidence that Renova® treats coarse skin, deep wrinkles, skin yellowing or other skin problems."

Renova® was approved by the FDA for the treatment of damaged skin to be used in conjunction with a comprehensive skin care regimen that included a sun-avoidance program. The effectiveness of Renova® "is dependent on other good skin care practices including avoiding direct sunlight, applying sunscreens, wearing protective clothing and using moisturizing lotions," according to the FDA.

Tazarotene, the Newer Trend in Vitamin A Treatments

Allergan, Inc. was given approval by the FDA in 2001 for the use of AVAGE® Cream that uses 0.1% Tazarotene, in the acetylenic class of retinoids (Vitamin A). It was approved under this trade name as a prescription medicine that may reduce fine facial wrinkles and certain types of dark and light spots on the face. This same formula has also been approved for the treatment of plaque psoriasis and acne vulgaris as Tazorac®.

The daily use of retinoids such as tazarotene is now approved by the FDA and only available by prescription as a treatment. Persons using AVAGE® daily receive the following information, which confirms why Total Oxidation Management is so important:

- The mechanism of tazarotene action in the amelioration of fine wrinkling, facial mottled hypo- and hyperpigmentation, and benign facial lentigines is unknown

- It should be used under medical supervision as an adjunct to a comprehensive skin care and sunlight avoidance program that includes the use of effective sunscreens (minimum SPF of 15) and protective clothing.

- Neither the safety nor the effectiveness of AVAGE® (tazarotene) Cream 0.1% for the prevention or treatment of actinic keratoses, skin neoplasms, or lentigo maligna has been established.

- Neither the safety nor the efficacy of using AVAGE® (tazarotene) Cream 0.1% daily for greater than 52 weeks has been established, and daily use beyond 52 weeks has not been systematically and histologically investigated in adequate and well-controlled trials

- AVAGE® Cream can cause birth defects in unborn children of women who are pregnant when they use the product. If you are a woman who can become pregnant, you must not be pregnant when you start using AVAGE® Cream, and you must avoid pregnancy while you use it.

- Avoid sunlight and other medicines that may increase your sensitivity to sunlight

- AVAGE® Cream does not remove wrinkles, repair sun-damaged skin, reverse skin aging from the sun (photoaging), or bring back more youthful or younger skin. AVAGE® does not work for everyone who uses it. It may work better for some patients than for others.

- AVAGE® Cream may cause severe irritation if used on eczema.

- Do not use if you take certain other medicines, Vitamins, and supplements that increase your sensitivity to sunlight. These include Vitamin A and medicines that are called thiazides, tertracyclines, fluoroquinolones, phenothiazines, and sulfonamides.

Laser Resurfacing or Laser Peels (Light Energy)

Laser resurfacing should be done for cosmetic reasons and only under the supervision of a medical doctor, usually a plastic surgeon or dermatologist, who has years of technical experience.

The word "laser" is an acronym for Light Amplification by the Stimulated Emission of Radiation. Lasers produce a specific wavelength of light that is beamed in pulsations onto the skin in controlled intensity and duration of the pulse. Within the laser unit, the beam of light bounces back and forth between optical mirrors and lenses. The light gains strength with each cycle and when it has reached the desired intensity, the light is released to create a quick burst of energy.

Most laser peels administered are for signs of aging including fine lines and wrinkles of the face, especially on the upper lip, cheeks, and forehead. Also peels are used for smoothing and tightening the eyelid skin, "crow's feet" around the eyes, removing brown spots and splotchy skin color, while minimizing scar appearance.

What usually comes with laser procedures is a very keen lesson to the patient on Total Oxidation Management. Even if the doctor or medical/salon professional did not call it Total Oxidation Management, their message is clear. Skin will oxidize much faster after a laser service. Do not allow your skin to oxidize after a laser service or the damage could be worse than the benefits of the service. Avoidance of all exposure to any kind of oxidation or free radical catalyst is absolutely necessary. That's Total Oxidation Management.

Ablative Laser Techniques

Ablative techniques, which infers cutting, removes the epidermal layer of the skin and the keratin protein and protective layers of the skin, heating the dermis layer to regenerate collagen. The intent is to allow the body to repair the "wound" created, resulting in newly formed, less damaged skin. There are three types of ablative laser techniques commonly used:

1) **CO_2** – Unlike the older carbon dioxide lasers, pulsed CO_2 laser emits a highly focused beam that enables the doctor to gently remove the skin's surface with a lower risk of scarring and other complications in properly selected patients. The skin affected generally heals over a two-month period.

2) **Er:YAG laser** – This laser procedure "produces energy in a wavelength that gently penetrates the skin, is absorbed by water (a major component of tissue cells), and scatters the heat effects of the laser light allowing doctors to remove thinner layers of skin tissue. It is used often for patients who have milder wrinkles or scars, or skin discolorations. Additionally, the Er:YAG laser is a more gentle touch for more delicate skin and may offer the advantages of reduced redness, decreased side effects, and rapid healing in or around a week."

3) **YAG Laser** – Developed in the last five years, this newer long pulsed laser delivers results that fit in between those of the CO_2 and the Er:YAG. According to the American Dermatology Association, "it provides more wrinkle relief and offers a reduced risk of scarring compared to both.

However, with less heat to the skin, results may not be as striking."

If you are considering a peel and laser as an option, ask your doctor if he or she is experienced in a non-ablative technique and if this technique could be effective for your condition. It provides a more Total Oxidation Management approach to the skin than the ablative technique.

Exciting New Non–Ablative Light Laser Therapies

Non-ablative laser techniques are more consistent with Total Oxidation Management since the procedure does not use oxidizers and does not leave the skin vulnerable to oxidation from the external sources that affect skin daily. The word non-ablative suggests the procedure does not cut and this procedure does not cause known damage to the surface epidermis layers like most peels, including the traditional laser.

These new light and radio frequency waves are referred to as photo modulation and are intended to by-pass the epidermis layers to reach the collagen producing cells (fibroblasts) in the dermis. One of the features of this relatively new technique is a cooling spray that helps protect the surface layers from being damaged. The technique is designed to damage the collagen production and cause it to contract. The theory is that this affect on the collagen producing cells will cause the body to repair the damage and within four to six months. The signs of aging become less obvious, with the upper layers of skin lifting and firming; however, it does not tighten older, sagging skin.

The target group for seeing the maximum results is thought to be those between their late 30's and mid-50's who have moderate damage. These procedures are not thought to be replacements for the more radical face lift, but instead for those who are showing the early signs of aging.

The healing time is less than traditional ablative procedures that cut, dissolve or burn away the surface layers. Still, it usually takes additional treatments to achieve the desired results. Many other medical devices now under development and many plastic surgeons are awaiting more data to determine the long-term results.

Another new non-ablative treatment is "photorejuvenation," which repairs collagen in the dermis, or deepest layer of the skin, while gently erasing signs of aging in the epidermis, or top layer of skin. Shorter pulses of light are delivered to the dermis; the collagen is injured and repaired. Photorejuvenation can reduce the signs of aging, including fine lines and wrinkles, sun damage such as freckles and irregular pigmentation, as well as redness and dilated capillaries associated with rosacea. The epidermis is rarely injured by this treatment, so there are no visible signs skin is undergoing this treatment.

Dermabrasion: Sanding Away Your Skin

The word "dermabrasion" implies what's involved in this technique, the removal of the skin down to the dermis layer using various physical crystals that break down the surface layers. This procedure is usually a one-time experience and does not require additional treatments like microdermabrasion. Dermabrasion, even under ideal conditions, can cause scarring, pigmentary disturbances, and skin texture changes.

For several weeks after a dermabrasion service, the affected area will be swollen, sensitive, and bright pink, which take months to subside. Normal activities may be resumed and the patient can be back at work in about two weeks, providing the skin is protected from any oxidation in the work environment and special attention is made to prevent the skin from any direct or indirect sun. However, the skin should not have any contact with the sun for up to one year due to the effect on melanin production. Swimming pools should be avoided for months due to the oxidizing affects of the chlorine, sun and wind. For three to four weeks the affected skin will likely experience a red flush when alcohol is consumed. The skin's pink complexion will take about 3 months to fade.

Doctors know the risks associated with this service, and as a result, most patients are fully aware when they leave the office that any exposure to the sun, cigarettes and oxidizers could lead to serious problems in the future. This is the reason a lifestyle of Total Oxidation Management should be adopted after dermabrasion.

Microdermabrasion

Microdermabrasion is less invasive than dermabrasion, but because it appears so gentle, the long-term risks are often ignored. Microdermabrasion of the skin can make the skin appear as if it were sandblasted. The process includes physically blasting the stratum corneum outer layers of the skin with sterile crystals to expose the younger proteins below. Usually, professionals recommend a series of four to six services every week or two over a two- to three-month period.

This particular procedure is often marketed as a "lunch-break peel," which implies that the invasion of the skin is minimized. A high percentage of microdermabrasion is conducted in areas such as Southern California, Arizona, and South Florida. Unfortunately, this is also where the exposure to the sun from just walking to the car after such a service is dangerous! Long-term effects can occur. Ironically, the service is done to remove age spots, and the fact is the service alone leaves the skin so vulnerable, that more age spots could actually be the result. Total Oxidation Management prior and following the service may improve the results and prevent many long-term risks.

Home Micro-Dermabrasion

No doubt you've seen them on TV infomercials and in beauty supply stores; the home microdermabrasion systems which have a light, abrasive sandpaper-like effect on the skin. Most have an abrasive on the surface of the device, and many are used in conjunction with a cream that contains abrasive crystals. The claims are usually associated with "removal of the surface layers to expose the more youthful skin below." This is another approach to physical exfoliation of the surface layers of the stratum corneum layer. Again, Total Oxidation Management is important if you choose this technique as a lifestyle.

Muscle Stimulation

The use of muscle stimulation machines has been a controversial issue in skin care for the past ten years. The theory suggests that electrical stimulation of a muscle can strengthen the muscle and might provide other benefits such as increased circulation that could lead to other benefits.

For small muscles in the face, I have found electronic stimulation the best and most effective method of keeping the muscles strong. The only device that I am aware of that is approved by the FDA is the Rejuvenique® Facial Mask that is manufactured by the Salton company. I find it especially useful in the improvement of "bags" under my eyes after days of travel. Combined with 2 steps in 2 minutes 2 times a day, the results are even greater.

Infrared-Light Therapy

Light therapy using infared spectrum wavelengths might be one of the more exciting technologies for skin treatments in the future. The concept is quite appealing and does appear to fit under the umbrella of Total Oxidation Management, since it does not require any invasion or radical peeling of the skin layers, and the wavelength of the light is not in the

UV spectrum that is known to increase free radical damage to otherwise healthy cells.

The biggest challenge presently is the limitation of the devices that are being used. Similar to muscle stimulation devices, the target is specific muscles and cells that would increase blood circulation and provide stronger, healthier cells. There are specific points in the face that could benefit, and to provide a thorough service, a balanced therapy needs to be applied to both sides of the face covering all key points.

However, the devices presently being used by skin professionals include a single wand or perhaps two wands that require a technician to apply, and therefore the benefits from the limited exposure to the infrared light is minimal. The benefits are achieved if all or most of the muscles and key points of the face are affected and the service is done with frequency.

Until there are devices that include more light exposure for more key points and the service is done with more frequency, the benefits are limiting and not really worth the investment. Still, look for advances in this technology.

Oxygen Therapy

Oxygen Therapy is another questionable trend in skin treatments

Logic would suggest that since we need oxygen to live, more must be better. I am not so sure, and I caution every person who has made a decision to allow oxygen therapy on their skin. Remember that oxidation involves the speeding up of the normal action of oxygen and increases the number of oxygen free radicals in the skin.

Day Spa Magazine is a respected publication in the skin care industry. In the February, 2003 issue, author Lisa Randazza states "Leading experts in the aesthetics industry have been arguing oxygen's value in skin care for more than a decade and are farther apart in their views than ever."

The reason they are further apart is that researchers are learning more and more about the danger of oxygen free radicals. Randazza does a great job of trying to show both sides, but most of the article is written from the perspective of the suppliers of oxygen therapy products. Their statements confirmed my basic opinion that the use of oxygen therapy (even though it sounds so healthy) is not a smart treatment service, should not be a lifestyle service, and could actually increase the oxygen free radical damage in the skin cells.

Three statements in the article demonstrate my serious concern and lead me to warn skin care professionals and their clients to think twice before they consider oxygen therapy, especially as a lifestyle service. Those statements refer to depletion of the acid mantle (lipids and proteins in upper layers) for oxygen penetration, use of hydrogen peroxide (oxidizer) for delivery of oxygen, and the need to create more energy in cells.

Oxygen therapy does not contribute to Total Oxidation Management. In fact, it is an example of Total Oxidation "Mis-Management." The benefits of oxygen therapies are more theoretical and less clinically proven. Until great benefits can be demonstrated to outweigh the obvious increase in oxidation potential, I cannot see the value of these services.

If You Are Still Planning Radical Exfoliation

As you've learned, any process that is intended to remove the surface layers of the skin must be taken very seriously. It is important to understand that any free radicals that might form without your knowledge during those days, weeks, and months following a chemical peel service are dangerous and will likely lead to extensive long-term damage.

If you are going to radically peel skin:

1. Know why you are peeling.

2. Know the depth of the peel.

3. Know what you should expect.

4. Know what responsibilities you have for caring for your skin following the peel.

If a radical peel process were done once in a lifetime, I would have little problem with it. Even if it were done once every few years, I would just caution the need for care during the days or weeks following the procedure. Unfortunately, this process has become a lifestyle for many, and they are combining it with other radical exfoliation procedures including Retin-A® or Retinol®, microdermabrasion, and even laser resurfacing.

Post Chemical Peel Care

I recently spoke with a massage therapist who works in a popular skin care salon who told me that three days after he had a "power peel" he went on an afternoon bike ride. He stated that for the following week, his skin looked and felt terrible. He stated he felt he had aged his skin instead of looking more youthful. In truth, he did age his skin, as those young, newly formed proteins that were exposed were not ready for any exposure to the environment and free radicals were forming that will cause serious damage to his skin in years to come.

It is advisable to have seven to ten days away from your job following medium-depth peels. Even light peels are tearing away the protective layers of the skin and require days or even weeks of absolute isolation from any sun, cigarettes, pollution and chlorine. Too often, the seriousness of the procedures of peels are understated to clients/patients. The comment, "Oh by the way, wear a sunscreen," is not close to the message.

This is the time that complete Total Oxidation Management must be adopted to avoid damage to your skin. Any exposure to oxidation that could result in free radical formation on that very exposed skin is dangerous and the damage could be irreversible, not apparent for months or years. In addition to not exposing your affected red skin to any direct or indirect sunlight for weeks or months, you must also pay close attention to any oral antibiotics prescribed.

The doctor cannot provide you a guarantee that you will not have problems because he and his staff cannot follow you around and provide you 24-hour advice. Safeguarding your skin after a chemical peel is your responsibility.

Be committed to a daily and intensive Total Oxidation Management lifestyle, including, the proper forms of Vitamin C and natural Vitamin E for at least six months following the peel, followed by the application of an SPF 15 sunscreen.

Stages of Healing

Three stages of healing are necessary during the recovery period following radical exfoliation to avoid complications:

First Two Weeks: Re-epithelization phase ("new" epidermis/ out layer of skin resurfaces the peeled or lasered skin). *Major Risk*: Infections.

Months Two-Four: Collagen remodeling phase (the upper dermis/middle layer of skin slowly heals and rebuilds itself) over two to four months (occasionally first six months). *Major Risk:* Scar Development (thickened or sunken scars).

First Six Months: The melanin pigment recovery phase is a risk because the skin color might never return to normal since the melanocytes are aggressively attacked and affected during the procedure. Lack of return of normal skin color can leave a light or white color which may be permanent, or a mottled clustered network of darker pigmentation can form. Often when this occurs, skin professionals immediately think of the need for another service to remove the pigment clusters. This practice can lead to permanent damage and discoloration. This affect on the melanin can leave the skin more vulnerable and create even more need for Total Oxidation Management.

The recovery of a "superficial" peel takes less time, but with the same urgent messages of protection. There should never be anything called a peel that is encouraged during lunch or any other inference to "come in when you have a moment." This is a serious treatment, and just walking to your car following the service is a dangerous risk.

If you peel your skin at home or administer peels to others, you must understand that the skin that is peeled should not be exposed to oxidizers, free radicals and any sunlight. That implies you should take off work for a week for a peel. Avoid even second hand smoke. A sunscreen on top of recently peeled skin is not the complete solution. Complete absence of UV rays on the skin is imperative. It is that serious.

Remember that for every layer you remove, it will take one to two days of new growth to return the skin to the protective layers that are considered somewhat safe. Total Oxidation Management is imperative during this period.

Summary of Resurfacing: Skin Deep Damage

The last ten years have created an explosion of exfoliation services in both doctors offices and in beauty salons, and many professionals and their clients are taking these services much too lightly.

Why do we think that nature has made an error and we need to remove the surface layers of the skin? As we've stated, most of these ingredients and devices advertise the removal of dead cels to reveal more youthful skin cells. Dead skin cells are not simply a "waste" product to be "trashed." Few people are realizing these "youthful" skin cells are just that — babies, or young protein cells (often referred to as "daughter" cells)— that are not ready for exposure to the environment.

The constant removal of the surface layers only leaves the skin more vulnerable to the environment.

Which leads me to the Hayflick Theory. Research by Dr. Leonard Hayflick in 1965 suggested that normal human cells cannot divide indefinitely. This limit of about fifty cell divisions is called the *Hayflick Limit*. The cells that have reached the Hayflick Limit may become sluggish, inefficient, and unresponsive to various signals from the body and unable to divide. Skin may become thinner, fragile, blotchy, and easily wrinkled.

Therefore, frequent radical exfoliation is risky because:

1. If you cut or burn yourself in the same place over and over (the result of a series of chemical peels), the affected skin tissue may become thinner over time and scar tissue may eventually form.

2. ANY sun exposure (UV-A or UV-B), cigarettes, or other oxidizers to the affected peeled skin that now has lost its upper protective layers of skin can transform previously healthy skin cells into unhealthy free radicals increasing potential problems with the skin in both the short term and long term.

3. The Hayflick Limit theorizes cells have limits on how many times they can reproduce. This could be a serious problem for those who choose to make chemical peels a lifestyle.

Remember, radical exfoliation should not be considered a lifestyle in skin care, and if you or a friend is considering a radical peel, it should be:

1) The last option for the treatment of the signs of aging since it is too risky. You might actually increase the signs of aging later due to the radical peel.

2) A treatment for a specific condition and never as a regular option for skin care since it is not cure; it is a dangerous violation of the protective skin layers.

3) A procedure that is a one-time only experience as opposed to an ongoing regimen.

4) Conducted by a skin professional who regularly processes radical peels.

5) Taken seriously with plans to remain at home and away from any oxidizing environment, and not go outside for weeks or months depending on the depth of the peel.

6) Stop smoking for at least seven to fourteen days.

Understanding Total Oxidation Management and employing it into your lifestyle, personally and professionally, could change the way you view peels and the wellness of your skin.

Normalizing exfoliation is a logical approach to skin care. After almost twenty years of experience and witnessing various conditions of the skin, I am confident that you can dramatically enhance your skin with a lifestyle Total Oxidation Management using our 2 steps in 2 minutes 2 times a day to normalize exfoliation.

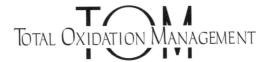

TOTAL OXIDATION MANAGEMENT

Conclusion

You Are Responsible for Your Skin

One of the most consistent lessons taught by religions worldwide is that we must take care of our bodies since our body is our "temple." And every day as researchers we are learning more about "our temple" and how it is built.

Your skin is your cover for the machine that is your body—your temple—the place in which you are living while visiting here on our oxidizing planet earth. You determine what to apply to your skin, what environments you expose yourself to, and what treatments you choose for your skin.

The oxygen that surrounds us is so necessary for our life functions. But as with everything, there is the Yin and the Yang, the good and the bad. For us to convert that precious element of oxygen to energy, an important "spark" of life, we must accept that with the good oxygen fuel comes the bad by-product, a free radical. As oxygen produces an action to create a substance, it can cause a healthy molecule to become dysfunctional and incomplete—and create a free radical that is missing an electron.

In short, oxidation creates free radicals and free radicals create dysfunctional molecules; unstable molecules lead to unhealthy cells that result in skin appearing aged.

You are now aware that...

You're Not Aging...You're *Just* Oxidizing!

The good news is you can help manage how fast you oxidize and slow many signs of aging with Total Oxidation Management, a wellness approach to skin care. "Wellness" is about making things last longer in their natural and original healthy form, not by stopping the activities you enjoy, but by simply shifting some behavior that may be causing you to age faster.

Total Oxidation Management is about being aware of how much you oxidizing every day. Changes in your lifestyle can be as simple as becoming aware of what is in your water that you use to shower. Or perhaps you will think twice about that convertible you dream about. Maybe the next time you go out to a sporting event, you will think about how long you might be exposed to the sun.

If you are a parent, you determine how fast your child will oxidize and show signs of aging in years to come. That precious little nose that is constantly being sunburned on the soccer field will likely develop into a serious skin condition when your child becomes an adult. You can take charge now by preventing the damage, and if there is previous damage, start today by teaching your son or your daughter that your goal is to stop free radicals from spreading to create more free radicals. Just as your child takes vitamins every day, they should be covered in the vitamins every day.

As soon as you realize you can start improving your life today by changing how you interact with the world around you, positive results will follow. Sometimes you will see immediate changes with Total Oxidation Management; other times it may take days, weeks or months, but you *will* see the results.

Living "In the Mode"

If you think you can't do anything about the effects of the environment where you live, what is in your water, and previous exposure to oxidation, you are making assumptions that are not true.

You can defend yourself by making choices that will prevent oxidation, such as limiting exposure to the sun, covering more of your body, but most important, stopping free radicals as soon as oxidation occurs. Once oxidation comes in contact with your skin, the most important proactive approach you can take is to cover yourself with ingredients that will stop the free radicals from forming on contact.

You can begin Total Oxidation Management today by applying a stable, 12% active L-ascorbic acid form of Vitamin C followed by a 5% natural Vitamin E product to stop oxidation and normalize free radicals. You may also supplement these vitamins with other good ingredients, sunscreens and better lifestyle choices. However, you want to know that while you are driving to work or playing outside, you have some defensive moves and some offensive moves you can take to keep fighting against oxidation morning and night.

Staying "In the Mode" with the application of these 2 vitamins in 2 minutes 2 times a day provides defense during the day against the harsh oxidation of the world, and works over night to help rebuild damaged cells and promote an improved appearance and healthier skin.

Changes You Can Make Now, No Matter How Old You Are

You might find people who have had similar conditions to you when you read the "Skin Conditions & Testimonials" that follow this chapter.

As you'll read, at any age and at any time, you can begin a lifestyle of Total Oxidation Management.

- If you are in your first twenty-five years of life, you can change your destiny and slow how fast you will age with Total Oxidation Management.

- If you are 25-50 years old, don't underestimate what is to come. Begin shifting your lifestyle and begin getting "In the Mode" today with 2 vitamins in 2 minutes 2 times a day.

- If you are 50-75 years old, you have begun to see free radical damage and you know how fast your skin can deteriorate. Don't despair and think you can cut off your skin and remove the damage. Slow down and understand you can reverse much of the damage by applying Vitamin C and Vitamin E to your skin — 2 vitamins in 2 minutes 2 times a day.

- And if you are in your fourth twenty-five years, congratulations! You have obviously oxidized yourself less than many of those friends who have passed on. With Total Oxidation Management and 2 vitamins in 2 minutes 2 times a day, you can still see significant improvements in your skin and on the age spots, bumps and lesions that are appearing on your skin from early damage from free radicals.

Only when the need for Total Oxidation Management becomes real to you will you shift how you view the world. You will make changes in your work, your play and your daily routine.

All it takes are simple shifts in behavior. And you will see the results!

Skin Conditions & Testimonials

Acne

We often think of acne as a problem faced by adolescents, but plenty of adults in their 20s through their 50s struggle with skin that is affected with the occurrence of acne either occasionally or on a regular basis. What might surprise you more about this common condition is the fact that the source of a breakout is a hair follicle.

Sebaceous glands in the hair follicle produce sebum. Sebum is an oily substance that, under normal conditions, travels up the hair follicle and out to the skin surface. As the sebum travels up towards the hair shaft, it encounters normal skin bacteria and dead skin cells that have been shed from the lining of the hair follicle. The greater the sebum production, the greater the likelihood that the hair follicle will become clogged as the sebum causes the cells of the follicular lining to shed more rapidly and stick together forming a plug at the opening of the hair follicle.

The mixture of sebum and dead cells becomes a pool for bacteria to grow in greater numbers than usual. The sebum, bacteria and shed keratin dead skin cells get trapped in the skin causing inflammation, swelling and pus, resulting in acne. The body responds to this bacterium pool by producing chemical defenders that can lead to the formation of free radicals as a by-product of the energy production. Acne lesions are most common in the areas of the skin where there is the greatest number of sebaceous glands including the forehead, chin and mid-back but acne can also flare-up on the shoulders, chest, neck, upper arms and scalp.

Hormones are the most common link to the causes for acne. The adrenal hormone DHEA along with increased levels of testosterone are associated with the exacerbation of severe acne. Testosterone, a potent male hormone, when oxidized is converted to DHT (djhydrotestosterone) by means of an enzyme called 5-alpha reductase. This is also the hormone linked to the loss of hair in both men and women.

Many women with acne are suffering from Polycystic Ovary Syndrome, a condition that involves the overproduction of male hormones, such as testosterone. If the acne is accompanied by changes in menstrual periods, fertility complications or weight gain, the acne might be linked to hormonal imbalance with high insulin levels in the blood and affect cravings that are difficult to control. A shift in diet to include many more vegetables and fewer carbohydrates might help in the control of this cause of acne.

Another hormonal link to acne is excess estrogen. An indication this might be a link would include other symptoms, including breast pain and headaches that might be accompanied by other skin complaints. Again, diet and supplements by the doctor might help regulate these hormonal imbalances.

Reports are indicating that the deficiency of progesterone might lead to the increased production of androgens (male hormones) that can result in acne conditions. The use of progesterone cream in some patients has been found to improve the appearance of acne.

Even infections caused by Candida and mucous membranes have been linked with an increase in acne. Even though this has been considered a weak link by many doctors, there are studies that indicate that managing the overpopulation of Candida might improve the appearance of acne.

Acne severity ranges from comedones, usually referred to as whiteheads and blackheads, to nodules and cysts. When sebum is trapped beneath the skin's surface, a closed comedone develops. A closed comedone is commonly referred to as a "whitehead." If the sebum is exposed to air, but is still stuck in the pore, it darkens into an open comedone or more commonly referred to as a "blackhead." Infection from comedones caused by bacteria leads to swelling, redness and pus. These infected cysts are sac-like lesions containing liquid consisting of dead cells, bacteria and white blood cells and nodules that are solid lesions that are the worst form of acne as they extend into the deeper layers of the skin. This form of acne may be very painful and can cause tissue destruction resulting in scarring.

Acne scars are usually classified into three categories:

1. Ice-pick scars are typically deep pit scars that can occur anywhere on the face.

2. Shallow, depressed scars appear to resemble shallow chickenpox scars.

3. Deeper, depressed scars cause deeper impressions usually found on the cheeks.

The age of the affected person also has led to categories for acne conditions:

Infantile Acne—As early as birth, infants can have mild acne on their faces, generally on the cheeks and occasionally on the chin and forehead. It is most common in male infants and is usually very mild. Fetal hormones appear to be the cause of infantile acne. Adrenal androgens, including excessive testosterone cause the increase in sebum in infants. Children with severe infantile acne tend to develop severe acne in puberty.

Adolescent Acne—Sebum production is controlled by the sex hormones. Acne usually develops when the body starts to produce the hormones called androgens. Androgens usually develop around the ages of 11 to 14, when puberty begins. As androgen production increases, and sebaceous glands enlarge, the inner lining of skin in the hair follicle changes. Normally, dead cells inside the follicle shed and gradually release through the surface. However, during puberty, dead cells shed more rapidly, that is, exfoliation is accelerated and the cells tend to stick together.

Adult Acne—While most people develop acne during adolescence, other factors can cause acne to occur in adulthood. These factors include:

- Environmental – High humidity can actually cause your skin to swell and pollutants in the air can also contribute to a higher incidence of acne in adults.

- Hormonal Cycle Changes – Women can experience intermittent acne associated with the hormonal changes caused by their menstrual cycles. Most of these breakouts occur one week prior to menstruation.

- Cosmetics – Whiteheads or closed comedones can actually be caused by cosmetics (such as foundations), night creams, and moisturizers composed of vegetable oils or oleic acid. Some cosmetic "cover-ups" actually aggravate the problem.

- Medications – the medicine that your doctor prescribed may cause your skin to secrete more oil than can be exfoliated normally, leading to an acne breakout.

- Genetics – Some people are born with a predisposition to acne. If your parents had acne as a teen, chances are you'll be more likely to also have issues with acne. While it occurs in all races, Caucasian Americans tend to be more affected by acne than African Americans, Hispanics of those of Asian descent.

Managing acne and the symptoms associated with the condition can be an ongoing process and therefore, it is imperative that your choice for managing the symptoms is a choice that can be incorporated into your lifestyle. Many traditional treatments are not lifestyle choices and can, in fact, adversely affect your lifestyle and your health, including:

Broad-spectrum antibiotics have long been used for systemic treatment of moderate to severe acne. Tetracycline, erythromycin, and doxycycline are all oral antibiotics used to treat acne and require monitoring by a physician for systemic side affects. Long-term use of antibiotics can increase the risk of antibiotic resistance in skin bacteria. A side effect of taking many antibiotics can lead to an increase in the skin's sensitivity to Ultra Violet light that can lead to an increase in the free radical damage of the skin that can lead to long term damage of the skin cells.

Hormonal therapies and corticosteroids may be prescribed for the treatment of severe acne but these methods of treatment can induce side affects with prolonged use. Isotretinoin, a retinoid (Chapter 14) has been recognized as the most effective drug available for cystic acne and acne that is resistant to other medications. However, a number of serious side effects are associated with isotretinoin therapy, including the potential for severe birth defects to a developing fetus. Thinning hair, joint and bone pain, depression, vomiting and nausea are some of the other less common side affects.

Chemical peels (Chapter 14) are often used to improve acne scars. The percentage of the acid used to peel the skin determines the depth of the skin layers the peel reaches. Chemical peels (glycolic, salicylic acid and 15% TCA) are used to remove the epidermis layers of the skin. These peels do little to improve ice-pick or deeper depressed acne scars where the damage is deep in the dermis layers of the skin. Recovery should include staying indoors void of any sunlight and avoidance of other oxidizers and cigarette smoke. Appearance affects include peeling, redness and flaking of the skin for a week following the procedure. Medium-depth and laser peels (carbon dioxide or erbium: YAG), peel away deeper layers of the skin however, recovery following these procedures can typically take weeks or even months and most people experience peeling, redness and flaking of the skin.

N-Lite® Laser has only recently been used for the treatment of acne. This light uses the yellow light energy to destroy bacteria. The light creates a chemical reaction by creating an oxidation reaction that is intended to kill the bacteria. Still, this does create free radicals as a side effect. Therefore, follow-up with the vitamin regimen of C and E is very important.

Dermabrasion is a common treatment used for shallow, depressed scars but the recovery can last months. The skin should not encounter any oxidation or sunlight for many months to follow as the skin layers that are intended to protect the internal layers have been removed with this procedure. Additionally, a series of microdermabrasion is now more popular than the deeper dermabrasion as the micro system does not go as deep. Still, this procedure does remove the surface layers of the skin and it should not be considered a lifestyle.

Collagen has been used by being injected directly into the acne scar and while there is no recovery time following this procedure, the results are not permanent and additional injections would be required.

The Wellness Approach

The wellness approach to Total Oxidation Management of acne can be a lifestyle choice and one that is easily incorporated into your daily life. Since acne involves bacteria, after cleansing the affected area, it is suggested that the astringent be used in conjunction with the 12% L-ascorbic acid form of Vitamin C in a non-oil based solution. The use of the 5% Vitamin E is only recommended after the acne is under control, perhaps after 28 days, to help minimize any scar tissue formation and even help reverse some of the appearance of scar tissue. This routine should be used morning and night to help normalize the natural exfoliation rate of skin to prevent sebum from getting trapped in the follicle, while killing the bacteria on the surface of the skin that can work its way down and be trapped in the sebum. The L-ascorbic form of Vitamin C is nature's own natural anti- inflammatory and can help reduce redness and inflammation associated with this condition while natural Vitamin E helps to prevent the formation of scarring caused by prolonged infection.

Our 12% *EC Mode® Vitamin C Serum* should always be used day and night following any other treatment service that removes the surface layers of skin as a treatment for acne. Even though it might sting a bit at first, since the pH is around 3, the ability of the vitamin to help prevent free radical from forming along with the suppression of visible inflammation can help in many ways.

The removal of scarring is one of the few conditions that I understand the use of the physical, laser, or sometimes chemical resurfacing techniques. As these services remove the abundance of lipids (oil) that can be the source of the sebum pool, there is logic to removing the layers IF there is disconfiguration of the skin. However, before any such radical service is attempted, it is important to attempt to manage the condition without invasive techniques, such as with astringent at night to help kill surface bacteria, 12% Vitamin C for the many benefits twice daily, and 5% Vitamin E after the first 28 days for moisture and helping to normalize any latent scarring.

Be aware that the 12% daily use of Vitamin C is not recommended to be applied at the same time as treatments that include any form of peroxide, which is an oxidizer intending to kill bacteria (it also can produce free radicals) since the Vitamin C will stop any oxidation activity making such a treatment useless. If any form of Vitamin A (Chapter 14) is used for acne treatment, it is recommended to use Vitamin C during the day and Vitamin A at night.

Additionally, gentle cleansing is always recommended prior to using the 12% *EC Mode® Vitamin C Serum* (a cleanser using AHA, e.g. glycolic acid is not recommended). Also, a clay mud masque weekly can help rid the pores of over-production of sebum without increasing oxidation.

Viki's Success

"I had adult acne, the hormonal, cystic type that was actually painful. It would flare up each month, especially along my jaw line."

As Viki knows, acne is a problem that many adults deal with well into their 30s, 40s and beyond. "My case was bad enough that I would see an esthetician every four to five weeks for extraction treatments just to help keep it under control," she said.

She's been a professional stylist for the past 13 years, recommending EC Mode®/Malibu Wellness products for her customers, especially before and after color treatments. "The water here in Ventura, Calif., is very hard, so for my clients, I use the *EC Mode® Fresh Start Shampoo* before and the *EC Mode® Emergent-C ReVITAlizer* after every color. My customers have noticed that their color lasts longer, and remains vibrant longer."

After having good results there, she decided to try the EC Mode®'s skin care line featuring *EC Mode® Vitamin C Serum*. It only took one month to see a difference in her acne condition. "Within that month my skin went from awful to beautiful! I had the type of acne that was deep under the skin, and I don't have it anymore."

Now, four months later, she has her skin routine down pat and in control. "I use the *EC Mode® Vitamin C Ancient Sea Clay Masque* once a week, and the *EC Mode® Vitamin C Serum* and the *EC Mode® Hydro-Driver* every day. I've been religiously using it for four month. When it runs out, I buy the next two kits, so that I never run out of it completely. I even have my 15 year old brother "In the Mode" and he uses the *EC Mode® Vitamin C Serum* to clean up his acne, too!

Viki says it's a whole new face staring back at her in the mirror, even when she uses a high-powered mirror. "I was looking at my skin in a 10x magnifying mirror and I don't have anything on my skin. Oh my gosh, there is nothing to extract! I'm just blown away by that. "

"My esthetician said 'What are you doing?' and I said that it has to be the Vitamin C. Now she wants to try it on her own skin."

Jenny's Success

Jenny has coped with acne for eight years. However, in her effort to treat her acne, she ended up actually irritating her skin and making her condition worse.

"When I went to the dermatologist, I was told that my skin looked exhausted. I tried so many products but nothing seemed to work. I have really sensitive skin and I started actually getting reactions to all the harsh treatments I was putting on my skin."

When the cream that the dermatologist recommended didn't work for Jenny, a friend of hers at work stepped in with some advice.

"When my friend suggested that I try the *EC Mode® Anti-Acne Kit* I didn't quite know what to think. I had actually seen the EC Mode® shampoo at the hair salon, but I hadn't checked out the skin care. I looked it over and it actually seemed too simple to me. I guess because I was used to seeing strong ingredients on the label. I read all the information about the Vitamin C and it made sense to me. So I tried it. And it made a huge difference. It worked."

Jenny uses all three of the components in the EC Mode® Anti-Acne Kit; the EC Mode® Facial Astrigent, EC Mode® Vitamin C Serum and the EC Mode® Hydro-Driver Moisturizer. "Before, my skin would break out with tiny bumps and it would feel tight and dry. But not any more. I've been using EC Mode® now for two years. And I haven't needed to go back to the doctor for my skin ever since!"

Age Spots, Keratosis & Comedones

The term "age spots" is somewhat of a catch-all. As we age, we begin to show signs of aging with dark spots, light spots, bumps, tags, crusty and other abnormal skin lesions. Still, the primary categories are usually related to either pigment changes to our skin or growths on our skin.

Pigment changes: Most of the pigment skin changes occur as a result of oxidation that occurs early in life. As explained in Ch. 11, melanocytes, which provide our coloring, are the sites where pigment is produced. Oxidation, especially from sun, can cause those melanocytes to be affected and create a condition later in life that causes a cluster of pigment or the other extreme, a complete loss of pigment, in an area of skin.

Other names for pigment age spots are liver spots (they are now known to have nothing to do with the liver), Lentigos, and Senile Lentigines. These dark pigment areas of the skin are pigment clusters that are very common after the age of 40. They often occur on the backs of the hands, on the forearms, shoulder, face, and forehead where exposure to the sunlight's radiation. They are usually harmless and painless, but they may affect the cosmetic appearance of the skin.

Keratosis is an abnormal condition of the skin where accelerated skin growth or pigment occurs, usually due to sunlight or another environmental condition caused previous oxidative free radicals in the skin layers. There are three most common types of keratosis:

1. *Actinic Keratosis* is a skin lesion resulting from free radicals, usually from too much sun exposure in early years of life. These lesions are the result of abnormal cell development in the stratum corneum of the skin. Even though they can appear at any time, they most often begin appearing after the age of 50. This abnormal condition is often the first warning sign of skin cancer. These growths should always be watched very carefully, since they can lead to pre-cancer and cancerous conditions.

2. *Keratosis Pilaris* - This condition appears often on the back side of the upper arm as prickly red bumps, much like a rash. Keratosis Pilaris is associated with people of German or Celtic backgrounds. It is an abnormal condition of the stratum corneum with little known long-term danger, with periods of "flare ups" when they appear more red and tender.

3. *Seborrheic keratosis* is a category of skin conditions that are the most common benign tumor in older individuals, but can form at any age. Seborrheic keratoses are brown, black or flesh-colored growths that can appear anywhere on the skin but mainly are found on the torso and temples. They can take on various shapes and sizes from wart-like growths, a flat network of pigment, or what many call skin tags.

They develop from the abnormal growth of the cells in the upper layers of the epidermis and are most often found on the skin that is over-exposed to sunlight. Some reports have linked these conditions to substances in the water such as arsenic. However, there is little connection to make such claims. They do appear usually upon exposure to sun or tanning bulb lights, but often do not appear until later in life when the free radicals have had time to continue to form abnormal cellular proliferation in the skin layers.

Seborrheic keratoses that appear to be web-like in appearance are referred to as reticulated and are usually found on sun-exposed skin and can also take on the look of large freckle-like spots. These spots do not all look the same as some are darker than others even on the same person. They usually affect lighter skinned people, but a variation is also found on dark skin that is often referred to as dermatosis papulosa nigra.

Comedones are small rough flesh-colored, white, or dark bumps found often on the face but also other parts of the body at the opening of a sebaceous gland or pore. These bumps are usually associated with sun exposure earlier in life and sometimes are confused with acne.

The Wellness Approach

Total Oxidation Management can help prevent and often diminish all of these conditions. As always, strict attention should be given to these unusual growths on the skin. However, unless a physician has determined there is cause for immediate removal, you may find that attacking the affected area twice a day—morning and night after every cleansing—with the freshly-activated ascorbic acid form of Vitamin C in at least a 12% solution followed by a solution of 5% natural Vitamin E can make a significant difference in the appearance and the discomfort of the condition.

These conditions are not diseases, and while Total Oxidation Management is not a cure, adopting this lifestyle and these vitamin-based products can help manage the condition and help it to remain more normalized.

Steve's and His Mom's Success

Dr. Steve L., of Clearwater, Fla., is no stranger to the world of vitamins—he consults in the field of chiropractic natural health and has been very active in this field for twenty-five years. During the past six years, he has participated in trade shows that feature health and skin care products. Over the span of his career, he developed the habit of sharing different vitamin products with his family, including his mother. "I'd send her all kinds of new things to try, so she's seen a lot over the years. But nothing has ever really impressed her to the point of specifically asking for a refill, except for one product: *EC Mode® Vitamin C Serum*," he says.

The skin on his mom's face was showing abnormalities from sun exposure, a form of actinic keratosis. She was reluctant to undergo treatment after seeing what her husband, Steve's stepfather, had gone through for the same problem. The doctor literally scraped deep in to the skin to remove all of her husband's affected cells.

Steve's mother was adamant that she did not want that done to the skin on her face. So she was especially receptive to her son's suggestion. Rather than resort to a more drastic approach, Steve gave his mom a bottle of *EC Mode® Vitamin C Serum* and *EC Mode® Hydro-Driver Moisturizer* to apply to her skin twice daily. A couple of weeks later, the spot on her nose was gone. When another case flared up on another part of her skin, she applied the products, and once again, had success. His mom was very pleased, but Steve wasn't surprised, since he had singled out this product line from all the others he saw at health and skin care trade shows across the country.

"You know I'm thrilled that it worked so well, but I wasn't shocked at how effective it was because I've seen this *EC Mode Vitamin C Serum* work so well with so many other people. Just by normalizing the skin cells with this fresh-dried Vitamin C, it seems like the cells are saying, 'OK, we can work again, we can get back to normal.'"

"My mom thinks it's great and she always lets me know when she's run out—she always ask, 'Can you send me more?' It's one of the few products she does that with."

Meanwhile, Dr. Steve follows his own consultant advice. "I use it, too. Every single day, right after shaving, I apply the *EC Mode® Vitamin C Serum* and the *EC Mode® Hydro-Driver Moisturizer*. Then at night, I wash my face and apply it again. It's in my own routine daily, because I know first-hand that this product stands out from the crowd!"

Broken Capillaries

Broken capillaries found in the skin are often the result of a genetic predisposition and occur most often in people with fair skin. The occurrence of broken capillaries is heightened with the lifestyle habit of over exposure to the sun (oxidative damage). Various contributing factors including consumption of certain foods or alcohol can exacerbate the redness in the skin usually caused by very small, dilated, blood vessels.

The most common form of treatment for broken capillaries is laser surgery. The laser light energy is absorbed by the red color of blood vessels and converted to heat, which seals the tiny blood vessels. Immediately the skin will become inflamed and bruising can occur which usually fades within 10-14 days. Sclerotherapy, an invasive method of treatment can cause pain, bruising and itching and hyper pigmentation of the skin. The expense of these treatments is not usually covered by medical insurance as they are considered cosmetic and if multiple treatments are required, the expense can be very costly.

The Wellness Approach

A wellness approach to broken capillaries has more to do with the inflammation and appearance of the condition than the total remedy. We have learned from many who use our fresh-dried vitamin technologies that they have minimized the appearance of broken capillaries and sometimes see them completely disappear.

A wellness approach is the use of our 2 steps in 2 minutes 2 times a day. Daily application of the 12% freshly-activated L-ascorbic acid form of Vitamin C, followed by a formula of 5% natural Vitamin E, can help minimize the inflammation associated with broken capillaries and improve the appearance of the skin where broken capillaries are usually found.

Lori's Success

For ten years, she's worn heavy-duty makeup under her eyes to conceal an imperfection that really bothered her. "I could actually see the bump in the skin, and I used the same makeup they use on burn patients to cover the red in the vein that showed through. It was really annoying."

Lori, of Davis, Calif., had a broken capillary under one eye that resulted in a bump that made her self-conscious. "I'm a sales representative to salons, and it's important to look good when I am presenting products. I had decided to get laser surgery to try to fix this, but then our company started representing EC Mode® products to salons and I attended a seminar with Tom Porter. I heard him talk about how the *EC Mode® Vitamin C Serum* had helped heal his scars on his face from a car accident. So I asked him if it might work on my broken capillary. He said he just didn't know, but to give it a try."

Lori decided to give it a try. "I think that when you use something, you can do a better job representing it, so I decided to begin using it every day. I put the *EC Mode® Vitamin C Serum* on in the morning and then the *EC Mode® Hydro-Driver Moisturizer*. And I just kept using it. The broken capillary just slowly, gradually faded. And now, I don't wear any of the heavy makeup anymore. I was actually shocked. The bump has gone down, too. My skin isn't red anymore; it's actually 97% better! What I like about this is the fact that it's natural. I'm very much into holistic health practices, so the fact that I didn't have to use laser surgery and was able to use vitamins is just great."

She also enjoys the new self-confidence she has. "I don't constantly look in the mirror anymore like I used to. First thing, I'd always check to see how it looked. Now, even in my family, no one notices it anymore. It's really cut down my makeup regimen, too."

Lori was so pleased with her own results that she's encouraged other members of her family to use the *EC Mode®* *Vitamin C Serum.* "My son has the traditional teenage acne breakout now and then. His skin will look red and inflamed and it's amazing how the *EC Mode®* *Vitamin C Serum* really calms his face down. It takes the red away."

Two different kinds of skin problems in one family, and one solution worked for both. "I tell all my clients about it. I mean, this isn't a scientific test, but it sure worked. And I'm thrilled about it."

Burns

A burn is an injury that damages and destroys skin layers. It can be caused by various sources, including a treatment, heat (scalding or thermal), electricity, chemicals, radiation or frost bite (freeze).

Electrical burns are the result of contact with live wires or unprotected electrical outlets, which vary with the intensity of the electrical current and how long the skin is exposed to the current.

Thermal burns are the most common type of burn, resulting from exposure or contact with a flame, hot liquids, hot objects, or from heat of a fire or steam with a temperature of above 115 degrees.

Chemical burns usually occur from contact with an acid or alkali. Many household and salon chemicals can cause a chemical burn, including:

- Peroxide (used in coloring, highlighting and perming hair)
- Sodium hydroxide (used in relaxing hair)
- Hydrochloric acid (used in toilet bowl cleansers and metal cleaners)
- Hydrofluoric acid (used in rust removers, tile cleaners)
- Phosphoric acid (used in rust proofing, disinfectants and detergents)
- Sulfuric acid (used in drain cleaners, metal cleaners and automobile battery fluid)
- Ammonia and phosphates (used in detergents and cleansers)
- Calcium hypochlorite (used in pool chlorinating agents and household bleach)

These solutions are strong oxidizing agents that, when exposed to the skin, can cause irritation or burning.

Freeze injuries are burns that are the result of extreme cold caused by weather (frost bite), or might be the result of a medical treatment, such as cryosurgery where the skin is "frozen" to remove layers of skin.

The severity of a burn is classified by the method and source of the burn and by the degree (see Chapter 14). The severity of a burn involves the depth of damage to the tissues of the body.

The Wellness Approach

The most common initial treatment of a burn is to clean the area to remove bacteria or debris that could lead to infection. Following this, we recommend putting it "In the Mode." Reports of healing following this application to the affected area have been very positive and the results have been dramatic. This application might tingle or sting, but with continued use, it will lessen as the affected area heals.

A wellness approach to chemical and thermal burns uses the 12% L-ascorbic acid form of Vitamin C and 5% natural Vitamin E to:

- Stop the oxidation of chemicals upon contact with the skin to prevent free radical formation.
- Help reduce inflammation and sensitivity, due to the natural anti-inflammatory properties of Vitamins C and Vitamin E.

Additionally, Vitamin C can help skin regenerate by increasing collagen synthesis (the connective tissue of skin), while Vitamin E can:

- Speed the healing process.
- Improve the formation of healthy tissue.
- Help modify scar formation.

For severe burns and especially those that are second or third degree burns, you should immediately consult a doctor.

Shirley's Success

The spots on her face were about the size of a dime, large enough for Shirley to not only notice, but also worry about. When she visited her dermatologist, his recommendation was to immediately remove them with cryosurgery, a procedure that uses liquid nitrogen to freeze (burn) the cancerous tissue and destroy it. She didn't think about the immediate after-effects, or how her skin would heal. Since she had traveled a great distance and they were going to scrape the tissue in order to test for skin cancer, it was suggested that she could save another trip in if they went ahead and removed them.

She wasn't prepared for what she saw when the doctor was finished.

"Now I had spots bigger than a nickel! I did panic. I could not believe it. The doctor had to go relatively deep on two of them since they were bigger than he originally thought. He said I may have scarring. Two of the spots immediately swelled and blistered and I thought to myself 'what have I done?'"

Shirley said the immediately results were painful as the swelling and blistering intensified. The dressing applied to the wounds in the office didn't help. So Shirley took matters into her own hands and tried to normalize her skin herself.

"I immediately went home and pulled out my *EC Mode®* *Vitamin C Serum* and *EC Mode®* *Hydro-Driver* and got relief. It was very soothing to the stop the heat."

She applied *EC Mode®* *Vitamin C Serum* and *EC Mode®* *Hydro-Driver Moisturizer* daily, expecting the healing process to take a long time. She was anxious to see how bad the scarring might be since one of the spots was "hollowed out," as she put it. "I thought that maybe in a couple of weeks it would be on its way to healing, but within days the one that had not blistered was completely gone. The other two were also better. The one that was the deepest was gone in a week and the worst one took no longer than a week."

The medical staff where she had the procedure was amazed at not only how quickly she healed, but how smooth and normal her skin looked.

"I had been using the *EC Mode® Vitamin C Serum* and *EC Mode® Hydro-Driver Moisturizer* for about a year, primarily because I had an age spot on my face that it was helping diminish. I have a tendency to scar anyway, so I am very impressed with these products. It was a lifesaver. I cannot be without it."

Chemically Peeled Skin

Chapter 14 focuses heavily on treatments using chemical peels such as alpha hydroxy acids. These acids have been marketed in the last decade as the greatest new trend in skin care. There is more confusion and more danger than people realize in the use of these acids.

Even though history mentions the use of sour milk and fruit in the improvement of skin complexion, there has never been such a wide usage of these procedures in the history of mankind as there is today. As indicated in Chapter 13, there is also a "great divide" in the acceptance and usage of these chemicals by both medical and salon professionals.

There is a good reason for this division. The overall usage of these products to radically peel away the surface layers of the face by dissolving the lipid oil substance (holding the protective keratin proteins) from the skin is dangerous more in the long term than in the short term. But even in the short term, these procedures are not without concern.

The "lunch time peel," the "complimentary peel," and other such marketing words indicate that the service is easy to administer. The extreme acid solution just dissolves away the "cement" holding the surface skin layers together. Simple, yet dangerous, since it can open the door for even greater oxidation and free radical formation in the skin cells, which leads to future problems often worse than the original problem.

Marketing slogans that advertise "Remove the dead cells to reveal youthful proteins" would be more accurate if it were worded "Remove the protective layers of your skin to reveal the new proteins being born that are not ready for any exposure to our environment." Yet, removal of the surface skin looks better weeks later without some of the pigment spots and fine lines that were visible prior to the service. However, skin has a memory and most of these signs of aging reappear, at which time, many think it is time to have another peel.

Chemical Peels Should Not Be a Lifestyle!

I am confident there will be a large increase in skin cancer victims in the next decade as a result of chemical peels. It is not the chemical applied; it is the removal of the protective layers and the dangerous vulnerability for weeks or months following. Even though an argument can be made that the skin should be covered with vitamins and sunscreens, I have witnessed hundreds of examples of clients who were smoking, cycling, golfing, and just walking from the store to their car unprotected.

What is worse is the use of these peels on clients who tan and who are advised that these peels are helpful to them. The combination of these lifestyle choices can lead to serious damage.

Additionally, it is important to understand that in the past decade, skin professionals have found that medium- to dark-skinned individuals often have hyper or hypo-pigmentation weeks or months following a peel. Caution should be taken on using chemical peels on anyone of Asian or African descent. And this leaves the most common procedure being conducted on the fair-skinned individual who already has free radical damage from years passed; and now, they are in more danger, since they have less protection during the weeks and months following their peel.

The Wellness Approach

Total Oxidation Management does not include the use of chemical peels as a lifestyle option. If such a procedure is administered, Total Oxidation Management is imperative following the procedure and then part of your daily lifestyle from that day forward. The vulnerability of the skin after such a procedure is dangerous. Sun exposure, cigarettes, pollution, and chemical oxidizers are all dangerous to that recently peeled skin and will lead to free radical damage that will become more visible in months or years.

Remain "In the Mode" covered at all times with Vitamin C and Vitamin E following a peel. If a doctor has recommended an ointment to prevent infection, use the Vitamin C under the ointment and the Vitamin E on top of the ointment. Once the ointment is no longer used, continue to use the *EC Mode® Vitamin C Serum* and *EC Mode® Vitamin E Hydro-Driver Moisturizer* at all times even when you feel the skin is fully healed. Additionally, a sunscreen indicating an SPF 15 should be used on top of the vitamins anytime the skin is exposed to the sun. And since the melanin has probably been affected by the peel, a suncscreen will be important to that skin forever.

Carol's Success

Carol is a nail technician in Pacific Palisades, Calif. who heard about Total Oxidation Management and fresh-dried vitamins from one of her clients. Carol has beautiful skin and is just approaching 30 years old. However, Carol developed a large hyper-pigmentation spot under her right eye that looked like a birthmark, which everyone was telling her was an age spot.

"This spot appeared when I had an AHA peel a few years ago. I was told this power peel of my skin would make my skin look even younger. First, the procedure made my skin very red and tender. But when it healed, it looked good. Then months later, I started to notice a small dark spot under my right eye. I went to my skin care specialist and was told I needed another peel. So, I had another glycolic peel."

Carol goes on to explain that after the second peel, the spot initially went away, only to reappear bigger. So, she was advised to have another peel. "I had another peel believing that the peel was removing my dark spot, not realizing that the peel was actually the cause of the dark spot. Months later the spot was as big as the size of a dime.

I finally went to a dermatologist. "I had never spent much time in the sun as a child, but I was being told the spot was caused by sun exposure from when I was young." The doctor prescribed "hydroquinone" to lighten or bleach the spot. And it worked. The spot was much lighter and Carol was satisfied until she was advised that hydroquinone is not a lifestyle product and it was only for a treatment of the spot. As soon as she discontinued the hydroquinone, the spot reappeared as dark as it had been before.

Make-up was Carol's only answer until a client suggested she try *EC Mode® Vitamin C Serum*. Carol's client suggested that it might take up to six months to see the spot fade, but that once it faded, she could remain on the product the rest of her life without concern.

Carol purchased the *EC Mode® Vitamin C Serum* and the 5% Vitamin E *EC Mode® Hydro-Driver Moisturizer* and began using the products. "I saw results the first day, and by the end of the first week, the dark spot was barely visible. I had clients commenting on my skin and I couldn't believe that in one week, the dark spot was not visible to my clients."

Now, Carol says "I'm 'In the Mode' everyday. It is clear that oxidation just in the air contributed to the appearance of the dark spot which was a result of the glycolic AHA peel." Carol advises her friends and her clients of what happened to her and does not recommend a "skin peel" to anyone.

Carol is "In the Mode" after every time she cleanses her face, which is morning and night. Her complexion is that of an 18 year old and she looks radiant. She continues to follow the trends and new technologies for skin. However, Carol knows when something works, and Total Oxidation Management on her face works...all day and all night long. Carol says she will never have another chemical peel in her life.

Elaine's Success

At the age of 37, years of chemical peels had left Elaine, from Phoenix, Ariz., with hypersensitive skin. After using most products, she would have breakouts followed by scarring. "I have religiously followed a good skin care regimen, at times sparing no expense," says Elaine. As a result of excessive exposure to the outdoors while she was growing up, the damage to her skin as she got older became more apparent.

"I have worked in the beauty industry most of my life and have had many corrective options available to me," says Elaine. To cover up the damage, "I began using makeup with more and more coverage. Eventually, I felt I had no choice but to seek out more aggressive alternatives.

She was told a polyglycolic peel would work, "which I did numerous times, with unsatisfactory results. At the time, Microdermabrasion seemed to be the most likely next step since I felt I had to take aggressive steps to improve my skin. While my skin texture began to show some signs of improvement, these series of skin resurfacing procedures seemed to make my face more sensitive and did not help normalize my occasional blemishes and scarring."

Then Elaine met Tom Porter. "I listened to his approach to normalizing the skin using Vitamin C and Vitamin E. It made me realize how simple the answer was. By normalizing my skin with the right form, percentages and delivery system of Vitamin C and Vitamin E, I could prevent breakouts that inevitably led to scarring and protect my skin from the environment."

Elaine began using the *EC Mode® Vitamin C Serum* and *EC Mode® Hydro-Driver Moisturizer* and within thirty days or so, "I could visibly see an improvement in my skin. Seeing these changes in my skin in such a short period of time, I am confident that continuing to use the *EC Mode® Vitamin C Serum* and *EC Mode® Hydro-Driver Moisturizer* morning and night will correct abnormalities of my skin and begin reversing cellular damage. This philosophy and approach not only makes sense but it is the answer and the results I have been looking for."

Cradle Cap

Infantile Seborrhoeic Dermatitis, also known as Cradle Cap, is a common inflammatory disease of the skin occurring in children under the age of one and usually within the first few months of life. Often, it appears in small, oily patches on the scalp, which flake away from the scalp. While the scalp is the area of the body most affected, Infantile Seborrhoeic Dermatitis can also appear in the eyebrows and eyelids. While this type of dermatitis looks unpleasant, it is not painful to the child and does not itch like Infantile (Atopic) Eczema.

Physicians may recommend plain bath oil to be added to your infant's bath water for mild cases of cradle cap; however, this recommendation will not prevent the adverse affects from the elements hiding in your bath water that can have on your infant's skin.

The level of chlorine in your bath water could far exceed the necessary requirements need in swimming pools to kill bacteria. This harsh oxidizer combined with hard water minerals can irritate your infant's skin and contribute to the condition. In severe cases of cradle cap, physicians commonly recommend a hydrocortisone cream (a steroid) to treat the symptoms. As mentioned in the Total Oxidation Management approach to Diaper Rash, steroids should not be considered until all other natural and more wellness approaches have been attempted.

The Wellness Approach

The wellness approach to Total Oxidation Management of Cradle Cap is a safe, gentle and effective way to help control and relieve the symptoms associated with Cradle Cap.

Fresh-dried vitamin crystals added to your infant's bath can neutralize the harsh oxidizing effects of chlorine that can irritate skin while preventing hard water minerals from further exacerbating the condition. Fresh-dried vitamins called *EC*

Mode® Vitamin C Inside/Out and EC Mode® Vitamin E Inside/Out are helpful in the bath water to normalize the skin. You'll see the most significant results when a *EC Mode® Scalp Actuator Normalizer,* which uses freshly activated Vitamin C, is massaged into the scalp for five minutes for three days in a row following the *EC Mode® Scalp Therapy Shampoo.* This approach in the proper percentage and delivery system applied to your infant's scalp can help normalize the exfoliation of the scalp layers and relieve the symptoms.

Shelly's Success

Shelly lives in southern New Hampshire. When Shelly's daughter was five months old, she started to develop cradle cap. Shelly's sister suggested her niece have an *EC Mode® Scalp Actuator Normalizing* salon service, since it is safe and uses freshly-activated vitamins. "We had one *EC Mode® Scalp Actuator Normalizing* service done on her, expecting to need more. Just one service in less than fifteen minutes took care of the problem. Now, I maintain her scalp using the *EC Mode® Scalp Therapy Shampoo,* which I find to be gentler than the baby shampoo I previously used. My baby is now eleven months old and the problem has never returned."

Renee's Success

"I heard so many different things from experts. Every single time my son got his hair cut the stylists would give me their opinion; that he wasn't getting the shampoo out when he rinsed, or that it was just shampoo build-up, or that he had dandruff, or eczema. And I tried everything to get rid of it," says Renee, a Cedar Rapids, Iowa resident,

Since birth, Renee's son Cole has had a very severe case of what's commonly called "cradle cap," a patch of skin on the scalp that flakes onto the shoulder. Over the past six years, she's tried everything to treat it from special shampoos to petroleum jelly, but nothing worked. In fact, some of the treatments were so harsh that they actually aggravated the skin condition and made his scalp bleed. "Cole knew he had a pretty bad case."

Renee decided to learn more about skin care and used the Internet to help her find products with vitamins C and E. "I did tons of research on the Internet and looked at so many brands, including Nu Skin®, Mary Kay®, Avon® and expensive Vitamin C serums. I found that a lot of vitamin C and E products were priced around two to three hundred dollars. If I had purchased the whole line, it would have cost $600!"

When her Internet search led her to www.WellnessSalon.com, Renee found the EC Mode® salon hair care with vitamin products not only for her son's scalp, but also for her own use. Furthermore, the pricing was within her budget.

"This was affordable! So I bought the EC Mode® skin care, body lotion, shampoo, hair thickener, and conditioner, too." The results for her son's hair and scalp were visible within a couple of weeks.

"The *EC Mode® Scalp Actuator Normalizer* absolutely worked. The cradle cap is completely gone. I keep the *EC Mode® Scalp Therapy Shampoo* in the shower, and now his brother uses it, too. It has really worked, and it didn't take long to see the difference."

While her son's scalp condition improved from the EC *Mode® Scalp Therapy System*, Renee noticed immediate results from trying the *EC Mode® Vitamin C Serum* on her face. "You feel like it's penetrating. My face actually feels tighter after I put it on."

Just a few weeks later, Renee started hearing compliments about her own skin. "People would say that I looked so much younger. I was just amazed with the results—for both of us."

"Thanks to the web site," Renee says, "it's convenient and easy to order."

Contact Dermatitis

Contact dermatitis is an inflammatory response of the skin caused by direct contact with an irritant or an allergen. The second most common type of contact dermatitis is caused by exposure to a material that one has become allergic or hypersensitive to.

The most common type of contact dermatitis is the result of contact with:

- Oxidizing chemicals (that may not be obvious or are hidden, for example, highly chlorinated water)
- Detergents, solvents or highly alkaline substances
- Poison ivy, poison oak, poison sumac
- Nickel or other metals
- Medications—especially topical medications
- Cosmetics
- Rubber
- Fragrances, perfumes

Contact dermatitis may also be caused by photosensitivity (exposure to oxidation caused by sunlight) when the affected area of the skin has been exposed to shaving lotions, sunscreen, perfumes and products containing coal tar.

The symptoms associated with contact dermatitis in the affected area are:

- Itching
- Inflammation (redness)
- Swelling
- Tenderness
- Lesions or a rash at the site of exposure which may ooze, drain or crust and may become raw, scaly or thick

201

Scratching a rash can spread the inflammation to other areas of the skin and lead to infection and potential scarring.

The Wellness Approach

A wellness approach to Total Oxidation Management of contact dermatitis involves the same defensive logic and a proactive offense using vitamins C and E. The name "contact" dermatitis makes it clear that something has to come in contact with the skin to cause it. Therefore, a defensive approach is to minimize the contact with something that oxidizes or irritates the skin. Covering it with a barrier lotion, such as *EC Mode® Hand Guardian*, is a lifestyle that may protect the skin from the irritant altogether.

Also, staying "In The Mode" takes the skin a step further to help conuter the oxidizing effects while normalizing the exfoliation rate and reducing inflammation. Using freshly activated L-ascorbic acid Vitamin C and natural Vitamin E can help reduce the symptoms associated with contact dermatitis. Remember no less than 2 steps in 2 minutes 2 times a day. And for most cases, attack the affected areas with additional applications after exposure to chemicals or substances that irritate the skin. Additionally, be prepared for light stinging for the first minutes after application the first days until the skin begins to be less irritated. The light sting is normal and you might go through an itching stage as the skin begins to heal.

Deborah's Success

"It wasn't only painful, it was embarrassing. The last thing I wanted to do was extend my hand to meet someone when my own hand was full of sores. Others might not want to even shake my hand, plus I was opening myself to infection. When you think about it, your skin is your body's glove and when I extended my hand with blisters, it was like having a break in the glove. I was subjecting myself to bacteria."

For just about all of her adult life, Deborah, who lives outside West Palm Beach, Fla., has struggled with a skin condition that has been labeled as many different conditions. She visited many doctors over the years, sharing her dramatic symptoms, only to receive varying opinions on the source of the problem and how best to treat the condition.

"My hands were cracked, blistered, itching, oozing, and dry. I had about a million different diagnoses – psoriasis, eczema, contact dermatitis, and stress. At some point, it just seemed like the doctors were all trying to say the same thing, 'I can't help you.'"

Nevertheless, a variety of treatments were tried. "I was given cortisone creams, injections, and oral medications such as Benadryl. I tried overnight gloves with cream and sometimes wore cotton gloves in the daytime. Finally, I saw a dermatologist and he said that all the cortisone creams were actually killing the skin."

By this time, her condition had also spread to her face. The dermatologist did an involved allergy test with patches that were to be worn for 48 hours to find out which chemicals might be causing an allergic reaction. The doctor thought she might have contact dermatitis, which would mean that her skin was reacting strongly to something touching its surface.

"I had been told by other doctors to choose products with 'urea' mentioned in the list of ingredients. Well, that ingredient is in probably 90% of the products out in the market now and guess what I was most allergic to? Urea!"

Deborah's introduction to Total Oxidation Management came at an instructional seminar for salon industry professionals in Atlanta last summer. When Tom Porter asked if anyone in the audience had dry, itchy hands – Deborah was the first to raise her hand to volunteer for an on-the-spot treatment of freshly activated *EC Mode® Vitamin C Serum*.

"I immediately felt a momentary tingling. At that point, my hands were itching and burning so much, that the tingling actually felt good! I instantly felt a relief in the tightness of the skin and I could actually bend my fingers without hurting them."

She bought her own supply of the *EC Mode® Vitamin C Serum* and the *EC Mode® Hydro-Driver Moisturizer* and began applying both products two or three times a day for a solid month. The results were dramatic.

"It took a full month for the healing, but about halfway through, at about day 12 to 15, I saw a huge difference; it was 80% better. My hands and face have literally lost 10 years! On my face, you can tell that my skin is hydrated, it's clear of the little rash and my pores look smaller. My skin on my hands finally looks like skin."

A side benefit that she is also pleased about occurred on her eyelid, where a skin "tag" (or excess flap of skin) had developed. "It used to be such a problem trying to put eyeliner on. One doctor had told me I would need surgery to get it removed. After day 10 of the *EC Mode® Vitamin C Serum* application, it literally fell off. I can put my eyeliner on straight now."

She looks back on all those years of skin problems and frustrating efforts with a fresh perspective and gratitude that finally her skin is normalized.

"I am so thrilled that I know about Total Oxidation Management and these products. I could have spent the rest of my life suffering, so I am thankful that I do know about this now. I'm not just treating the symptoms; I'm actually participating in the cure for my condition. You can't just treat the symptoms; you need to treat the cause."

Dandruff – Itchy, Flaky Scalp

Dandruff, eczema and psoriasis are conditions of the scalp that affect millions of people. Even though these conditions are often regarded as "disease" by the FDA and FD & C, these conditions are sometimes nothing more than an abnormal exfoliation rate and the result of exposure to the elements of the water used at home.

Chlorine and calcium are two elements that are found in water that can make a simple scalp condition an abnormal and problematic condition. Some of the treatments recommended for these conditions include cortisone, prednisone, zinc pyrithione, tar, salicylic acid, and other ingredients that might be as much a problem as the problem itself.

The common symptom of these scalp conditions is usually the abnormal exfoliation rate of the protein layers of the skin (Chapters 11-12). This is not just a genetic condition and therefore often these symptoms are not a disease at all. What is in your environment could be causing the aggravation and before medications are used, simple wellness solutions might improve the feel and appearance of your scalp.

The Wellness Approach

A condition of the scalp should be considered abnormal exfoliation, and the first treatment should help normalize it with fresh-dried vitamins in the salon, in the doctor's office, salon or at home.

The most important aspect of Total Oxidation Management of the scalp is to actuate or jump start the normalizing of the exfoliation rate with the use of freshly activated vitamins. As this is a safe and harmless approach to managing conditions of the scalp, it becomes a lifestyle option. When the condition flares up, attack it with a scalp massage of freshly activated vitamins for at least seven minutes and then daily use of a scalp therapy shampoo and conditioner that are effective and do not make the condition worse If a patch of skin continues to be a problem, apply *EC Mode® Vitamin C Serum* and *EC Mode® Hydro-Driver Moisturizer* to the area, since it is more concentrated and safe even for an infant.

So often when people respond that our shampoo and conditioner are effective and they have not used any of our freshly activated vitamin products, I know that the problem was the shampoo or conditioner they were using. The use of the *Scalp Actuator Normalizer* at least monthly, the *Scalp Therapy ReVitalizer* monthly and the use of the *Scalp Therapy Shampoo* and *Conditioner* daily might be the lifestyle solution that provides you constant relief with ingredients that are completely safe.

Marcia's Success

It was an outbreak the whole family experienced after they moved into their new home in Indianapolis—sores on the scalp. They suspected it was something in the water; Marcia says it's known for being very hard, but the plumbing setup in their house didn't have enough room for a water softener.

Luckily, her cousin, who was in cosmetology school, had a suggestion – try the *EC Mode® Dandruff/Eczema* kit that includes the normalizing and revitalizing system that also often eliminates the appearance of eczema and dry flaky scalp conditions made worse by what is in the water. She used the products and began using the *EC Mode® Scalp Therapy Shampoo* and *EC Mode® Scalp Therapy Conditioner* daily.

Her cousin had learned about using C and E to manage the effects of too much calcium in the water. "Art bought it for us at the beauty supply store and brought it home. We tried it and it worked. It took the sores right away. This is just the best!" said Marcia.

"When we ran out of the EC Mode® products, I used what was in the shower. We had the *EC Mode® Scalp Therapy*

Shampoo for two weeks before it ran out (our whole family was using it). So, once again, we had problems with the hard water. The bumps on our scalps came back. My husband also started getting really dry flaking on his scalp."

Without the usual beauty supply source, Marcia wondered how she could fix this hard water problem again. "Well this time, when I was just about out of the *EC Mode® Scalp Therapy Shampoo* when I just happened to notice that on the bottom of the bottle there was the web address, www.WellnessSalon.com where I could order through the Malibu Wellness network of salons. Finding www.WellnessSalon.com was very good."

Marcia's family has found the answer to their hair, scalp and skin issues and now purchase their EC Mode® products from the salon right on the Internet.

"My three sons even looked for it at home, they actually came into my bathroom and stole it for their shower it worked so well. By rotating between the *EC Mode® Scalp Therapy Shampo* and the *EC Mode® Revitalizing Shampoo*, we keep the problems at bay."

Diaper Rash

Diaper rash is a condition that is usually associated with red inflamed skin with a prickly rash on the skin of an infant during the time a diaper is worn. A diaper rash is usually a combination of factors, including exposure to urine, feces, moisture, friction, and perfume or other chemicals used in disposable wipes. Often parents are told the problem is that they do not change the diaper often enough. As that can lead to compounded problems, diaper rash can occur with regular changing cycle as well.

One factor that doctors and other professionals have neglected is the water that the infant is bathed in. We underestimate the effect chlorine (used in our water systems to kill bacteria) has on a sensitive infant's (and everyone's skin for that matter) skin. Additionally, in water that contains high levels of calcium (over 100ppm can be a problem for some; however, hardness levels can exceed 200ppm or even reach 600ppm in some parts of the country) the problems to the skin can be significant.

The Wellness Approach

Steroids should be a very final alternative and should not be considered unless all natural and sensible approaches have failed. All efforts to normalize the condition with a shift towards Total Oxidation Management might prevent you from having to use any treatment that could have undesirable side affects.

You want a solution that is a lifestyle so that undesirable treatments do not have to be used on your family's skin. By using fresh-dried vitamin crystals in the infant's bath you might immediately begin changing the appearance of the skin to a more normal condition. If a patch of skin continues to be a problem, *EC Mode® Vitamin C Serum* and *EC Mode® Hydro-Driver Moisturizer* is the next action to take since it is more concentrated and still safe for even an infant.

Elena's Success

Elena lives in Castaic, Calif. and is a mother who faced a problem that most moms deal with at some time with their babies – diaper rash. "When my son, Maximillan was about six months old, the problem really started flaring up. He would cry and cry, and especially if pre-moistened wipes were used at diaper time. I tried so many creams before taking him to the doctor. Finally, we did take him to see the doctor, because he had also developed eczema on his back and on the backs of his arms."

However, Elena wasn't thrilled with the professional recommendation from the physician. "The doctor prescribed a steroid cream, which I really didn't want to use on my baby. But we had such a problem, so I tried the steroids for about five days. However, it didn't help."

Elena heard Tom speak on the subject of Total Oxidation Management using *EC Mode® Vitamin C Inside/Out* and *EC Mode® Vitamin E Inside/Out* bath crystals. She had suspected that the hard water in her home that was high in calcium deposits had caused some of the problems. She felt that using the Total Oxidation Management for skin issues and water issues at the same time made sense.

"It was pretty easy to use. At Maximillan's bath time, Elena simply sprinkled a little of the fresh-dried crystals from each of the shakers. "There was no stinging, no crying. And the other amazing thing is the fact that the diaper rash relief appeared to be immediate! I was surprised that the suffering from diaper rash was stopped and then all appearances of the eczema on his arms and back began diminishing completely in just three days."

"I'm finding myself using more and more of Total Oxidation Management and Malibu Wellness products for my own use and even for my husband. I just purchased the *EC Mode® Vitamin C Serum* and *EC Mode® Hydro-Driver Moisturizer* in the

EC Mode® Wrinkle-Less Kit for my own face, and my husband is using the *EC Mode® Optimum Hair Growth Tonic* for his own hair and scalp. And I bought the *EC Mode® Hand Guardian* for our hands and feet."

But she hasn't forgotten the little person or the problem that helped her discover the importance of regular use of fresh-dried vitamins C and E every day on his skin.

"My girlfriend's baby was also struggling with a bad case of diaper rash and I shared some with her, and now she uses it on her child, too!"

Eczema of the Skin

The term eczema refers to many different skin conditions that are characterized by inflamed, irritated, itchy skin that can become moist, ooze and can result in scaling patches or fluid-filled bumps.

According to the American Academy of Dermatology, atopic dermatitis is the most common form of eczema. It affects millions of people every year, and surprisingly, infants and children are more prone to this condition than adults. Atopic dermatitis occurs when inflamed cells move upwards toward the skin's surface and cause itching, redness, and swelling. What triggers the cells to overreact or exfoliate too rapidly and become inflamed is not conclusive, yet it does have many of the symptoms of free radical damage.

What is known is that exposure to an oxidizing environment, such as chlorine and even calcium in water used to bathe, can cause the symptoms to flare up. The condition is exacerbated during the winter months when skin is exposed to the oxidation of cold, dry winter air combined with overheated rooms. Other triggers that worsen atopic dermatitis are oxidizers found in cleaning solvents and other chemical compounds that you might be using every day. While there is no known cure for atopic dermatitis, the symptoms of this form of eczema can usually be controlled and relieved with a wellness approach.

The Wellness Approach

The Total Oxidation Management wellness approach to treating eczema (dermatitis) is a non-irritating, non-invasive approach to relieving and controlling many of the symptoms and improving appearance of this condition.

Our wellness approach may either replace the need for certain medications, including steroids, or complement some of these medical therapies. Placing your scalp "In the Mode" with EC Mode® freshly activated vitamins and shampoos/ conditioners that do not contain many ingredients that might irritate the scalp or skin. This approach could be helpful in the weaning off medications that are not recommended as a lifestyle.

For the skin and for the scalp, take a bath instead of a shower every day for a week using Vitamin C and Vitamin E fresh dried *EC Mode® Inside/Out Crystals*. Second, apply *EC Mode® Vitamin C Serum* followed by *EC Mode® Vitamin E Hydro-Driver Moisturizer* to the affected area at least twice daily. Some users express immediate relief and for others it may take up to 28 days to see the improvement in the appearance of the skin.

For the scalp, use the L-ascorbic acid form of Vitamin C in the *EC Mode® Scalp Actuator Normalizer* and the *EC Mode® Scalp Therapy ReVitalizer* to help provide relief to the flaking, inflammation, and appearance of the condition. Along with the *EC Mode® Scalp Therapy Shampoo* and *EC Mode® Scalp Therapy Conditioner,* this approach is especially beneficial for those people bathing in water high in chlorine or calcium and other elements that might affect the skin condition.

Alexis' Success

"Her skin was hard, red and calloused. It wasn't even as soft as leather, it was more like an elephant's hide. She doesn't sweat, so she lacks moisture. There is no 'cure' for it, so the doctors didn't know what to do about it."

Kathy, who lives in Lakehurst, New Jersey, is talking about her five-year-old daughter, Alexis. "I took her to several dermatologists, and had allergy testing done at the University of Pennsylvania. She was even hospitalized at one point."

Alexis suffers from the "elephant hide" callous condition called Ichthyosis Vulgaris which covers over 80% of her body. Kathy stated that only one percent of all the people in the world have this condition. The symptoms of cracked and bleeding skin, especially on her hands and feet are commonly associated with atopic dermatitis (commonly known as eczema).

"Her fingers would crack and bleed. The bottoms of her feet bled so much that she would come down the stairs walking on her knees. She was making do with what she had. It's hard to remember how many ointments they put her on. Cetaphil®, Eucerin®, and then the topical steroids they prescribed were awful because they made her scream so loud from the burning. The people from across the street could hear her. Next the doctors tried an oral steroid prescription for 30 days, but that had so many negative side effects and it made her hyper."

A friend of Kathy's owns a hair salon and suggested that Alexis try the EC Mode® Vitamin C and E line of products. Kathy began by sprinkling *EC Mode® Vitamin C Inside/Out and Vitamin E Inside/Out* crystals in her daughter's bath water. Alexis noticed that there was some stinging in the beginning, but everything that touched her skin caused that reaction and this wasn't nearly as painful as the steroids.

Next, Kathy activated and applied the *EC Mode® Vitamin C Serum* to her daughter's skin followed by the *EC Mode® Hydro-Driver Moisturizer*. "The first time I got it, we put the *EC Mode® Vitamin C Serum* on three times that day. This was the first time she slept through the night and the itching stopped. To go in and see her resting is worth all the money in the world."

In just a month, Alexis was like a different child. "Her skin is now looking beautiful. You can see the healthy skin that is forming. You'd never know she had a problem. I have seen kids on the *Maury Povich Show* with this condition, but now you wouldn't know my daughter has this problem. It is very emotional. When I took her to the doctor he said, 'I don't know what to do.' Well, now I do."

Kathy applies the *EC Mode® Vitamin C Serum* in the morning before Alexis goes to school and her daughter makes it through the entire day without itching. At night, another application is done after she bathes with the *EC Mode® Vitamin C Inside/Out* and *EC Mode® Vitamin E Inside/Out* crystals in her bath.

Kathy is taking her EC Mode® products to her daughter's physicians to show them the difference this treatment has had on Alexis' skin. She hopes that the doctors will, in turn, let other patients know about Alexis' story.

"My daughter will never be without the EC Mode® Vitamin C and E products in her life. Until God cures her, gives her radiant skin on her own, we have Malibu Wellness in our lives. It's my daughter's miracle. I'm so blessed."

Victoria's Success

Wendy's three-year-old daughter, Victoria, was diagnosed with severe eczema when she was just one year old. "She was just a mess. Her skin was so red and dry that she would scratch it with her fingernails to the point it would bleed. I had to keep her nails really short to make sure she didn't scratch," said Wendy.

Her daughter's physician wrote a prescription for hydrocortisone. When that didn't work, the next prescription would be for a stronger steroid cream.

At the time, Wendy worked for a distribution company that serviced professional hair and skin salons. She heard about Malibu Wellness and decided to try *EC Mode® Inside/Out Vitamins C & E* in her daughter's bath water. Previously, Wendy had limited her daughter's baths to just once a week, because they dried her skin so badly.

Victoria's bathwater was lightly sprinkled with the fresh-dried vitamin crystals (E & C), and then followed up with the *EC Mode® Hand Guardian* lotion.

The results were immediate. "It really is a 'see it to believe it' thing. I've recommended this product to so many people, but they just can't believe that one product line could do this much. I bet I've told about a hundred people about it."

Bathing in the EC Mode® normalized Victoria's skin, and the *EC Mode® Hand Guardian* helped seal in moisture to support the skin's healing process.

Today, her daughter's skin looks normal, and Wendy does not worry about keeping her daughter's fingernails severely trimmed. Her mom has her skincare regimen down to science.

"Our *EC Mode® Inside/Out Vitamin C* travels from the bathroom to the kitchen!" says Wendy. Not only are Victoria's baths sprinkled with the Vitamin C, Wendy uses this same product (Inside/Out just like the name implies) to keep Victoria's peeled apples fresh for her snack at pre-school.

She also uses the EC Mode® *Vitamin E Inside/Out* in the bathwater, and mixes a little of the *EC Mode® Vitamin C Serum* into the *EC Mode® Hand Guardian* to apply directly to her skin after her bath.

Victoria turns four this year, and the days of dry, red, cracked, and bleeding skin are behind her. Her mom vows that her daughter will not go through the agony she used to endure ever again.

"If I were stranded on a desert somewhere and was allowed to only take one thing with us, it would have to be my EC Mode® Vitamin C. I would be lost without this product."

Dry Skin & Irritated Hands

The most common irritation on skin is the hands. This is due to the amount of contact our hands have with substances in our environment. And the most common cause of dry, irritated hands is oxidation.

Dry, chapped, cracked, irritated and inflamed hands would fit most appropriately under the "contact dermatitis" category. This is a perfect example of "cause and effect" that was discussed at the beginning of the book. Something caused the effect on the hands.

The hands have an extra layer of skin called the stratum lucidum. Nature has provided this extra layer of dead protein as an extra padding which protects this exposed skin. However, it is still skin and can have reactions to simple oxidation. As discussed throughout this book, oxidation can come from many sources. Just the constant washing and drying of your hands can lead to oxidation. The wet/dry cycle speeds up oxidation. Detergents with some fragrances or colors might irritate the skin that allows the oxidation to compound the problems.

Most often, if you look around, you can discover the oxidation that is affecting your hands. In many occupations, oxidizers are all around us. For example, a construction worker would not realize that the concrete is calcium based, and that along with the water cause the hands to become very irritated.

Nurses are subjected to chemicals and the constant cleansing and drying of their hands. The worst occupation might be hair professionals, who make most of their money using oxidizing chemicals such as peroxide. Combined with the constant exposure to water, often with minerals and chlorine, hair professionals' hands are in the greatest danger when they are rinsing the chemicals from the hair. This explains why so many complain that they wear gloves but still have problems.

Usually, they remove the gloves while rinsing, thinking all the chemicals are gone. This is actually the time most of the damage is done to their hands.

For years, I have attempted to explain this to dermatologists who treat hair professionals' hands with steroids, including cortisone and prednisone. In fact, steroids are not a lifestyle choice and should be one of the last approaches to consider. Once dermatologists stop to consider that the problem is the oxidation of the hands, the dermatologist can assist the professional in understanding Total Oxidation Management and use ingredients, such as freshly-activated Vitamin C, to help stop the oxidation and apply a barrier on the skin and also stop the oxidation throughout the day and provide therapeutic benefits at night.

The Wellness Approach

Remember, Total Oxidation Management is about defense and offense. The defense involves being mindful of your activity and perhaps shift some behavior to minimize the exposure of oxidizers to the hands.

The most important defensive aspect of maintaining healthy hands is to use a barrier cream that will guard against the air, water, and chemicals that can irritate the hands. That would be like wearing an invisible glove, but still being able to have complete use of the hands.

The most important offensive play you can do is to use the L-ascorbic acid form of 12% Vitamin C, followed by a layer of solution with 5% Vitamin E , both in the morning and in the evening to stop oxidation and promote healthier cell functions.

Rod's Success

When Rod cuts hair on stage, there's a spotlight, huge audiences of adoring stylists, dancers, and lots of loud rock 'n roll!

Besides operating his own salon called "Images by Rod & Co." in Rantoul, Ill., he's an international platform artist with Sexy Hair Concepts® and travels the globe as the main attraction for important hair shows. He wields the tools of his trade almost like the main character in the movie "Edward Scissorhands".

The finished cutting edge haircut he brings to his models elicits "oohs and aahs" from the professionals in the audience who clap and whistle like fans at a rock concert. In that rock concert mode, he teaches stylists the latest techniques, with skilled hands that have sculpted thousands of haircuts.

Today, he's a star in the business, but about 15 years ago, he almost had to quit the profession that has brought him fame. The hands that masterfully cut, nearly failed him because of the exposure to oxidating chemicals , such as peroxide, used in hair coloring/bleaching solutions and perms.

"When I got my cosmetology license and first started working with colors and especially perms, my hands would break out terribly. I would have open sores that cracked and bled, like dermatitis. It actually began when I was in school to get my cosmetology license. I wasn't sure at all that I could go on," he said.

For awhile, he thought he might have to give up the part of his profession that included using color and perm chemicals. He went to physicians for help, but found no relief in the steroid creams they prescribed. "When I would go to the doctors they would treat the symptoms with creams for dermatitis. But they didn't know how to fix the actual problem, because they didn't understand the oxidation processes that were going on in the salon and how to manage them."

That changed when Rod found Malibu Wellness. Once he understood Total Oxidation Management, he had control of his hands and most of his challenges that he had with the chemicals in his salon. Rod learned about Total Oxidation Management and how to use this new concept in the salon to insure the health of both his clients' hair and his own skin.

"Tom Porter and Dr. Ault taught me about Total Oxidation Management. They taught me how to treat the problems, not the symptoms. First, I began using Malibu Wellness *EC Mode® Crystal Gel Normalizer* before and after my services to prepare the hair then stop the oxidation that was in the water and in the chemicals. I learned that water itself is an oxidizer due to the chlorine and then you just add more oxidation with peroxide. You're in "total oxidization" until you use the *EC Mode® Crystal Gel Normalizer* to stop the processing. Without it, well, it was like putting layers of Velcro® over my hands! Over time, at the end of the day, they just eat at your skin. You can stop oxidation on the client's hair and on your skin with the fresh-dried vitamins in the *EC Mode® Crystal Gel Normalizer*."

Rod began teaching Total Oxidation Management to clients and other professionals and to this day, Rod is still a part of the Malibu Wellness Salon network. Once he began getting his skin "In the Mode," the improvement in the condition of his hands was incredible. He added more products to his own regimen by including *EC Mode® Hand Guardian* lotion.

"Hand Guardian is like an invisible glove, it's really something else that's great in the Malibu collection. The Malibu Wellness collection complements the other products we have in our salon and onstage with Sexy Hair Concepts®. I use them both all the time. In fact, because I do a ton of color all the time, I truly believe that a stylist can not be a good colorist unless he or she understands the principles of oxidation and uses *EC Mode® Crystal Gel Normalizers* to control it. Unfortunately, I believe that 90% of all hairdressers out there still do not understand how to control oxidation. When their clients leave the salon, their hair is still oxidizing."

Today, Rod Sickler makes it a point to emphasize information about managing oxidation when he teaches stylists in his salon and at his shows. He remembers how badly his own hands hurt from exposure to oxidizing chemicals and passes on what he has learned to others in the business. "I hoped that I've saved the skin of other professionals, as well as, of course, helping the clients' hair!"

To this day, Rod makes sure his own skin stays "In the Mode." As he puts it, "I still use *EC Mode® Hand Guardian* every day. And right before I go to bed, I continue what I've been doing for more than ten years by putting the *EC Mode® Vitamin C Serum* and 5% Vitamin E *Hydro-Driver Moisturizer* on my face. People sometimes guess my age to be 10 to 15 years younger!"

All in all, not a bad thing for a rock and roll stylist!

Teresa's Success

When Teresa finished cosmetology school in 1989, her hands were a mess from all the chemicals she used when applying color and processing perms. "I was in terrible, excruciating pain every time my hands touched plain water. The skin was cracked and broken," says Teresa, who is from Madison, Minn. "If you could have only seen how deep the blisters and cracks were; 85% of the skin on my hands and on my wrists was just raw. I would use gloves at the salon and try all kinds of lotions, but one time I woke up in the middle of the night with my finger bleeding from the ring cutting into my finger. It was so bad that I had to get my wedding ring cut off. It was that extreme."

The doctors told Teresa she would need to leave the profession and enter a new career because there was no way she was going to be able do hair. They said she was allergic to permanent and tint solutions. But it was her life's dream to be a cosmetologist since she was a little girl. "I've been told that I'm stubborn and I guess because of that, I wasn't about to give up on that dream. So I took my state boards anyway, and received my license and accepted a job at an in-store salon at the JC Penney department store. But since this was a full service salon that did color and perms, I didn't know how to make it work. Luckily, for me, the manager of the salon told me about a product called *Malibu 2000 Crystal Gel Normalizer.*"

The manager said to her, "What if I told you that you will be able to do colors and perms? Give yourself a month working here with this Malibu products. If in a month you can't handle the chemicals, you can just do haircuts."

When Theresa first started working at the salon, she did all the Malibu Vitamin C Crystal Gel Treatments for clients. "That put my hands in the Vitamin C all the time. At the end of the first week, I was better! So, I just continued to use the *Malibu 2000 Crystal Gel Normalizer* on all my chemical service clients and on my hands and all of the shampoos. I realized that I was not allergic to perms and colors, but that my skin was just over-oxidized!

"I've learned to keep my hands 'In the Mode.' My scar tissue on my hands is gone now. You'd never see the signs now. I make sure that I stay 'In the Mode' with the Vitamin C on my skin all the time.

Poison Ivy

We have all been taught, at some point in our lives (usually as children) what poison ivy looks like. The typical poison ivy leaf is made up of three leaflets which are reddish in color and joined together by a common stalk. While we are all familiar with poison ivy, according to the American Academy of Dermatology, approximately 85% of the U.S. population will develop an allergic reaction if exposed to poison ivy, poison oak or sumac.

Poison ivy is caused by exposure to urushiol (pronounced oo-roo-shee-ohl), a chemical in the sap of poison ivy, poison oak, and sumac plants. Urushiol is found inside the plant; however, the stems and leaves of the poison ivy plant are very fragile and therefore are easily damaged by wind and animals which can cause pressure to the leaf resulting in the release of the urushiol. Pets, clothing and tools can also carry the sap or oil that contains the urushiol to the skin.

Poison ivy is a form of contact dermatitis. Most people develop sensitivity to urushiol after several encounters with the poison ivy plant. Sensitivity can occur after being exposed one time. While a reaction from a first time exposure is rare, signs of the reaction in the form of a rash may take up to seven to ten days to appear on the skin. The urushiol must penetrate the skin through the surface stratum corneum layer of the skin to deeper layers where the cells can experience an adverse reaction in less than one minute.

Less of a reaction usually occurs where there is the extra stratum lucidum layer (Chapter 11) such as in the soles of the feet or palms of the hands. Exposure to the urushiol oil causes an allergic reaction resulting in a rash, itching and blisters. The severity of the symptoms depends on how much of the urushiol oil a person is exposed to and their level of sensitivity. Only 1 nonogram (a billionth of a gram) is needed to cause the rash on some people.

Contrary to popular belief, rubbing the rash will not cause it to spread to other parts of the body beyond the affected area nor can it be spread to another person. The rash can spread only if the urushiol oil has been left on the hands.

However, the rash might appear to be spreading if it appears slowly as opposed to all at once. This is caused either by the urushiol being absorbed at different rates in different parts of the body or due to repeated exposure to objects that were contaminated by the urushiol sap. For this reason, cleansing the affected area as soon as possible could help to prevent the urushiol from attaching to the skin, according to Hon Sum Ko, M.D. an allergist and immunologist with the FDA Center for Drug Evaluation and Research.

According to Dr. Ko, cleansing may not stop the initial breakout of the rash if more than ten minutes has gone by: however, it can help to prevent further spreading of the rash. If you can't cleanse the affected area quickly enough or if your skin is so sensitive that cleansing doesn't help, inflammation (redness) and swelling will appear within 12-48 hours. If the urushiol is trapped under the fingernails and blisters are broken from scratching, infection can develop, as with any wound, and scarring can be more likely.

The Wellness Approach

Treatment for poison ivy depends upon the level of exposure and therefore, the severity of the reaction. Immediately after rinsing, get "In the Mode" by applying a solution of no less than 12% Vitamin C followed by a solution of 5% Vitamin E to help normalize the activity. The use of soap and a scrub or exfoliant are not recommended since they could spread the urushiol. Hot water is not recommended, as it can cause increased inflammation and swelling.

Staying "In the Mode" will not only help normalize the free radicals that are forming, but also help reduce the inflammation and prevent scar tissue formation. These 2 steps in 2 minutes at least 2 times a day has been reported to help prevent the spreading and many of the symptoms associated with poison ivy, poison oak and poison sumac.

Cindy's Success

Cindy who live in Randolph, Mass., had no idea why her arms were burning up with an itchy rash, but she was lucky to have a previously scheduled appointment with the doctor. She was shocked with the instant diagnosis – poison ivy.

"I've never had poison ivy in my whole life, and I don't like to do yard work very much, so I was shocked." But she did remember that she had trimmed some bushes in her yard, so she knew that perhaps that had led to the run-in with poison ivy. "All I knew was that this was the most horrible itch I've ever experienced in my entire life. I couldn't stop scratching it, yet the more I did – the more it itched," she says.

Her doctor prescribed a cortisone steroid and gave her some Benadryl® to take when she got home. However, before doing that, Cindy stopped by her daughter's house for a short visit. When Cindy showed her the rash, her daughter knew just what her mom needed. She told her mom to try the *EC Mode® Vitamin C Serum* that she was using to treat her own rosacea condition. Cindy was skeptical.

"I told my daughter that nothing was going to help. I also told her the doctor gave me some Benadryl® to take at home. I was absolutely convinced that there was no cream or lotion that was going to put out this fire. But my daughter was persistent and she wouldn't take 'no' for an answer. After we went back and forth for awhile, I said I'd try it."

By this time, both of Cindy's arms felt like they were on fire with the poison ivy rash. She took the bottle of *EC Mode® Vitamin C Serum* and applied some to each arm, followed by the 5% Vitamin E *EC Mode® Hydro-Driver Moisturizer*. Cindy felt better immediately, much to her shock.

"All I can tell you is that it worked. It just calmed the fire and the itch right away. It was just amazing and I really did not believe it would work. But it did. My daughter kept saying, 'I told you.' She seemed to enjoy being right, and her mom being wrong," Cindy laughs.

"That's okay, because my poison ivy felt a lot better."

Psoriasis

Psoriasis is an abnormal condition of skin cells called kera-tinocytes (Chapter 5). Keratinocytes are formed in the lower epidermis of the skin and move toward the surface as new cells are generated from below (Chapter 11). While the cause of psoriasis is unknown, it is often a predisposition that might be passed through genetics. Recent discoveries indicate that immune cells, called T-cells, appear at the sites of increased keratinocyte activity and might be increasing the production of free radicals which certainly trigger inflammation of the skin.

As a result of this inflammation, skin exfoliation speeds up and becomes abnormal. Due to this rapid exfoliation, cells stick together and build up on the skin, causing scales that can become quite large and might even bleed. Because kera-tinocytes cells make up most of the epidermis, any part of the body covered with skin may be affected. However, the most common areas afflicted are the scalp, lower back, elbows, knees, groin, genitals, nails and skin folds.

Symptoms of psoriasis vary in the shape and pattern of the scales and in severity. In mild cases, people may not even re-alize they have psoriasis. In severe cases, the symptoms can be very irritating and painful and can cover a vast area of the body.

Traditionally, treatment of psoriasis has ranged from those that have mild side effects to invasive drug treatment that can cause potentially dangerous side effects. Steroids (cortisone creams and lotions) are often prescribed to help temporarily clear or control the condition. This method of treatment is not a lifestyle choice, since side effects of these stronger prepara-tions can include changes in skin color, bruising, thinning of skin and dilated blood vessels.

Abruptly stopping the steroid can result in a flare-up of the disease, and after months of this form of treatment, the condition may actually become resistant to the steroid preparation. Long used for the treatment of psoriasis of the scalp, coal tar-based shampoos are also not a good lifestyle choice and can be harsh and irritate the scalp if scratched. Retinoids (prescriptive Vitamin-A related gels), often prescribed alone or in conjunction with topical steroids, are also not a lifestyle choice as side effects can include dry skin, elevation of lipids in the blood and bone spurs. Oral retinoids should not be used by women who are or may become pregnant within three years of use due to the risk of birth defects. Anthralin® is a topical medication that can cause irritation and staining of the skin and clothes. Cyclosporine® and Methotrexate® are oral drugs that may be prescribed when all other methods of treatment have failed.

Invasive methods are known to cause potentially dangerous effects to internal organs and require close medical monitoring. And finally, light therapy and PUVA® (combination of the drug Psoralen® and the use of UV-A light) are often used in cases of severe psoriasis or when other methods of treatment have failed. These methods of treatment used over a long period of time can increase the risk for free radical damage to the skin, including premature aging and pigmentation changes, as well as, the risk for skin cancer.

The Wellness Approach

While there appears to be no known cure for psoriasis, the wellness approach uses Total Oxidation Management with freshly activated L-ascorbic acid form of Vitamin C and a 5% concentration of natural Vitamin E to help relieve many of the symptoms associated with psoriasis, including:

- Normalizing the natural exfoliation rate of the skin.
- Reducing inflammation and redness.
- Relieving itching.

A Total Oxidation Management approach to psoriasis can be a lifestyle choice since it is non-invasive, non-irritating and does not cause any side affects. Many people who suffer from psoriasis have informed us that the use of EC Mode® products has provided them relief and the appearance is remarkably improved, allowing them to stop strong medication.

Danielle's Success

"Last year I was diagnosed with psoriasis, which has been a challenge for me, especially because I am in my early twenties," says Danielle of Seattle, Wash. "In the beginning, I was using ointments and special bulbs to reduce the problem; however neither worked the way I felt it should. Soon after, I started using the *EC Mode® Vitamin C Serum* twice a day accompanied with the *EC Mode® Hydro-Driver Moisturizer*, and the psoriasis that used to make me so self conscious is nonexistent! This is an absolutely amazing skin product and I will use this product for the rest of my life!"

Ana's Success

Ana of Watsonville, Calif. is thrilled that finally, she can wear a ponytail. Or tuck her hair behind her ears and show off a new pair of earrings. Since she's been a young teenager, she's struggled with a skin condition that left the skin on her head and scalp looking red, raw and feeling tight. One other symptom was especially problematic—flaking.

"When I was a teenager, people would notice it and comment that I had dandruff flakes showing. And I'd explain that this is a skin condition, not dandruff on my shirt. My skin could get tight and itchy, too. If I scratched at it, it would bleed."

"I developed psoriasis when I was about 13 or 14 and at first, my mom thought that all the dry skin behind my ears was from me not washing my hair thoroughly enough or that dried hair spray was causing the problem. But it also developed other places besides the ears, like on my scalp, on my forearms, and spots on my chest and back. So I went to the dermatologist."

The doctor's treatment was not pleasant. "I had to buy tar shampoos and ointments that were prescribed. One ointment had a steroid in it and that provided a little relief but I didn't want to stay on a steroid forever. And these products smelled awful. They were also expensive, since my insurance didn't cover it."

Believe it or not, later on, her best solution was pregnancy. "While I was pregnant, the psoriasis really cleared up on my scalp. So my doctor thought that maybe the prenatal vitamins were providing something in them that was working for me, something I was lacking." After she had her baby, Ana continued taking the prenatal vitamins, hoping that provided the answer. Unfortunately, the psoriasis returned. "My doctor actually joked that maybe I should just stay pregnant all the time. I said 'no thank you' to that."

Ana's long-term solution involved camouflaging her psoriasis with her hairstyle; covering the spots that showed on her head with her hair and wearing long sleeves to cover my forearms. After graduating from Beauty College, she became a store manager for a company that sells products directly to professional stylists. That's when she began hearing a lot about different products from the manufacturers' representatives who came in and held workshops on their particular brands.

"I kept hearing from various product experts at the store that their brand works on psoriasis. Then I'd try it and it wouldn't work, so I became skeptical. And I admit that I was still skeptical when Tom Porter came in and held a workshop about Total Oxidation Management using *EC Mode*®'s *Vitamin C Serum* and *EC Mode*® *Hydro-Driver Moisturizer*. He kept saying, 'You have to try it," and he actually came over with a bottle of EC Mode® Vitamin C Serum and had me put it on my skin right then and there. So I started using it. Right away, there was less flakiness. The area that used to be bright pink—now you see the real color of my skin. It's not pink anymore. My family was the first to notice it. My mom said, 'What happened to the psoriasis on your forehead?' She thought I was using a new kind of camouflage."

Ana's results after just three months have answered her initial skepticism. "I'm very thrilled and impressed. This actually works! I've been 'In the Mode' now for three months and you should see the condition of my psoriasis, or should I say 'try to see it' because it is amazing! I'm no longer ashamed of letting people see my forehead and forearms. I am also exposing my ears now, because that's the other place that was so bad. I'm able to show off my ear lobes and my skin doesn't feel dry and irritated, either. It feels very soft. I will stay 'In the Mode' for life."

The reason Ana probably had no skin conditions while she was pregnant likely goes back to the early research on Total Oxidation Management when it was found that the body retains its high concentration of Vitamin C during pregnancy rather than it being excreted. So now, instead of living in a pregnant mode, Ana can live in the EC Mode® and find relief for the rest of her life.

Tom's Success

Tom, of East Hartford, Conn. has been plagued by psoriasis on his back and right thigh since he was a boy, visiting every type of specialist and taking both internal and external medications to try and clear it up. "Nothing, and I mean absolutely nothing, worked," says Tom.

"On most days I have experienced open pustule bleeding and pain. At times, the sores would bleed right through my clothes, which is humiliating to anyone, especially in a business situation! I finally settled for a topical ointment provided by my doctor and decided that I would have to 'live with the mess.'

One day, Tom's wife encouraged him to try her *Wrinkle-Less Kit* from EC Mode®. "I said no, I was afraid to stop using the medicine. My wife pointed out to me that (the medicine) was not working anyway, so what did I have to lose? I agreed to a one-month trial period for the sake of peace and harmony.

"Two times a day, I began using *EC Mode® Vitamin C Serum* and Vitamin E *EC Mode® Hydro-Driver Moisturizer.* No one was more surprised than me to find the bleeding stopped after one week! By the end of the month, I was almost cleared up! I couldn't believe my eyes. The results stunned me.

"It has been over one and half years since I began using the product, and I am free of sores and bleeding discomfort, and even my scars are healing. My doctor is amazed! I just want to say thanks to Malibu Wellness for making such a wonderful product."

Reconstructive Surgery (Before & After)

Reconstructive surgery is selected by patients for many reasons, but usually to alter the appearance as a result of an accident, birth abnormality, or to help reverse signs of aging. Most reconstructive procedures involve the cutting of skin. Even though this procedure might appear invasive, it usually does not include the removal of the upper skin layers. Therefore, this becomes a condition that is more similar to wound healing than exfoliation services.

Reconstructive surgery is more consistent with the principles of Total Oxidation Management than radical peel services. For example, I would recommend an eye lift by a plastic surgeon before I would recommend a chemical or laser peel. Most reconstructive procedures involve the cutting away of layers of skin. While chemical peels completely remove the protective cover of skin, reconstructive surgery usually involves cutting and stitching, meaning the lower layers of skin are less exposed to the outside environment. Strictly following the advise of the surgeon is important, and as soon as possible, begin the use of Total Oxidation Management after the surgery.

The Wellness Approach

Prior to Reconstructive Surgery

Even though some physicians may question whether there is any benefit to applying Vitamin C and Vitamin E prior to the surgery, I highly recommend it. Doctors usually agree there is no harm done; but little clinical research has been conducted on the use of these two vitamins prior to surgery. However, there is little clinical evidence that just moisturizing prior to a procedure offers significant benefits.

Many people who have used Vitamin C and Vitamin E simultaneously prior to surgery have had such positive results during their healing process that they believe the healing process is faster and the scarring is minimized. Of course, these same people are using the 2 steps after the procedures; therefore, it is difficult to separate the finding. However, it is highly recommended to begin using the L-ascorbic form of Vitamin C and a 5% solution of natural Vitamin E prior to the procedure.

Following Reconstructive Surgery

Before beginning the use of the freshly activated L-ascorbic acid form of Vitamin C, do a "spot-test" on a section of your treated area to determine sensitivity. Initially, you will likely experience a tingling sensation, which will diminish within seconds. Begin using the freshly-activated L-ascorbic acid form of Vitamin C in a concentration of 12% to your entire treated area when the level of sensitivity on the spot-test area is tolerable. Consistent use of the L-ascorbic form of Vitamin C will result in diminished sensitivity due to the development of newly formed skin cells. The sooner your treated area is able to tolerate the slight sensitivity, the sooner you will accelerate the healing of your treated area.

Begin using a 5% solution of Vitamin E, following application of Vitamin C, after the sutures are removed to hydrate the deeper layers of skin, continue to speed the healing process and help inhibit the formation of scar tissue. This combination should be applied morning and night after cleansing and may be used in conjunction with any antiseptic recommended by the doctor. Always consult with the doctor regarding caring for your skin following this procedure.

Mary Lynn's Success

"I'm a sun freak; I'll admit it. I've been one all my life, and I'm paying for it now."

Mary Lynn lives on the beautiful, sun-drenched coast of South Carolina. Unfortunately, her sun worship days are over. Two years ago a freckle on her face was diagnosed as melanoma. The scar that it left was incredibly deep.

"By the time the doctor finished with the surgery on my face, I had a crater in my right cheek about the size of a measuring tablespoon. It took seven digs to get all of the melanoma. I was horrified when I saw it," she said.

Her dermatologist sent her to see a plastic surgeon, Dr. Marcelo Hochman, in Charleston, to have a reconstructive procedure. "After the sutures were removed, Dr. Hochman introduced me to EC Mode® and explained that by using the *EC Mode® Vitamin C Serum* and the *EC Mode® Hydro-Driver Moisturizer* twice a day, I could help reduce the scarring. I massaged it into my skin twice a day. He told me it would help diminish the scar in time. He did say that it would take time. In about six months, I was able to tell a big difference. First of all, the scar was not as red and it flattened out, it wasn't as raised up. Without makeup, you can still notice the scar, but it has really diminished the redness. When I wear makeup, though, you cannot see it at all. Friends who didn't know that I had the surgery can't tell. The Vitamin C and E have made a huge difference."

"I am really sold on these products and I am not that way about many products. But this scar on my face would not be as camouflaged if it weren't for the *EC Mode® Vitamin C Serum* and other EC Mode® products. I will never be without it. I also use the *EC Mode® Silk Sunscreen* under my makeup and on my neck."

Mary Lynn hopes that her story will serve as a fair warning to other women and young girls about the dangers of skin cancer, beginning with her own family. "I want to get the *EC Mode® Wrinkle-Less System Kits* for my daughters. They are also sun freaks, and I'm afraid they're following in my footsteps."

Rosacea

If you look like you're constantly blushing, chances are you may have a very common condition called "rosacea."

Rosacea gives the appearance of persistent "flushed" cheeks or sunburn. It usually affects the center of the face, but can also affect the chin, forehead, ears, chest, and back. Over time, the redness becomes ruddier and visible blood vessels may appear.

Rosacea is a chronic condition that can be very disruptive to one's life. An estimated 14 million Americans are affected by at least one symptom of rosacea and many more are not aware that they have the condition.

As the condition progresses, small pimples, which resemble acne can develop, although the actual comedones (white or blackheads) do not form. Other potential signs of rosacea are burning or stinging of the face accompanied by itching or a feeling of tightness. Eye irritation gives the eyes the appearance of being bloodshot or watery, a condition known as ocular rosacea. Rosacea should be treated, because as it worsens, the skin may thicken and enlarge from excess tissue, most commonly on the nose. This more severe condition of rosacea is called "rhinophyma."

Sometimes spicy foods, extreme temperature changes and can aggravate or trigger rosacea. The actual cause of rosacea is still not scientifically known, however, the following are theories related to rosacea:

- The sebaceous glands have more sebum than normal, which builds up on the skin and forms a flaky film (similar to cradle cap on babies).

- Rosacea might be related to how often and how intensely people blush. When you blush, a large amount of blood flows through vessels quickly, which causes those vessels to expand quickly to handle the flow. When this occurs, the skin's immune system tries to control this inflammation by sending more blood supply to the area which can then cause broken blood vessels.

- Rosacea might be related to the bacteria known as "Helicobacter Pylori." This bacteria is known to be in the plaque residue found on teeth but also has been found in the stomach where it might be the cause of ulcers.

The Wellness Approach

By using vitamins C and E in the correct formulation you can:

1. Cleanse deep into the mouth of the follicle to help prevent sebum from building up.

2. Normalize the natural exfoliation rate of the skin to help prevent clogged pores.

3. Gently cleanse skin with mild cleansers that prevent irritation to dry, sensitive skin.

4. Replenish moisture to dry, flaky skin.

5. Soften skin.

6. Help protect skin from UV radiation that can cause inflammation.

7. Help protect skin against harsh oxidizers in the environment (air, sun, and water) that can irritate and aggravate the symptoms of rosacea.

Lisa's Success

Lisa is actually in the salon and skin care business. She's a manufacturer's representative to salons and spas, so she's had access to just about every product available for sale over the counter. However, nothing she tried was working on her condition, so she decided to consult with dermatologists.

"I've always had a little pinkness to my skin, but for the past four years, I've had a lot of redness, hard bumps under the first layer of skin and it just looked like I had sunburn all year around. I tried a couple of doctors and they put me on different prescriptions. I tried Metrogel®, Benzocream®, and one dermatologist wanted me to take an oral antibiotic. I even had a prescription for a steroid cream for the itching. They said I had rosacea," Lisa said.

There were two problems with the products they prescribed; they did not work and they actually irritated her skin. "I've tried everything from the basic ten dollar cream to the most expensive department store creams and everything aggravated it or made it worse."

Relief came unexpectedly at a seminar she attended on behalf of the salon distribution company that employed her. Lisa attended a workshop on the EC Mode® Vitamin C and E product line taught by Tom Porter.

"At that first seminar he described rosacea and asked if any of us had this condition. At the time, my face felt like it was on fire. It was like I had been in a tanning booth or something. I raised my hand and right there on the spot, Tom Porter mixed up a fresh batch of his *EC Mode® Vitamin C Serum* and I put that right on my face. Within five minutes, the heat was out of my face. By the end of the day, the redness was gone."

Her daily skincare routine now involves at least two applications of the *EC Mode® Vitamin C Serum* and *EC Mode® Hydro-Driver Moisturizer*. And her rosacea is under Total Oxidation Management.

"Certain things will set rosacea off, like spicy foods. But on a daily basis, my face is not red like it was before. It's been a year and I have not been back to any of my doctors for my skin condition."

She also swears by the *EC Mode® Silk Sunscreen* too. "I love the sunscreen. It's the best ever. I'm really sensitive to dyes, colors, but this really feels good on my skin after I use the *EC Mode® Vitamin C Serum* and the *EC Mode® Hydro-Driver*."

Her own experience with the product line and her skin has helped Lisa feel good about representing this product line to salons and spas in her region. "I like to sell from the heart, and when I find something that I believe in, then I can represent it. I really believe in what this company stands for."

Skin Cancer & Skin Growths

*"The incidence of melanoma is rising faster than
any other type of cancer. 51,000 new cases of invasive
melanoma are expected in the U.S. this year."*
The University of Texas, M. D. Anderson Cancer Center, 2003

Oxidative free radicals can lead to the formation of cancer. Cancer can occur when free radicals form in cellular molecules in such large numbers that the DNA is actually affected. If the free radicals are allowed to continue to multiply within cells, the cancer can often spread or metastasize either deeper and in other regions of the body.

Researchers have separated skin cancer into three different categories:

Basal Cell Carcinoma	Develops in the Basal layer of the epidermis. Doesn't metastasize (spread to form in other cells). Curable upon early detection
Squamous Epithelium	Made up of squamous epithelium. Can metastasize or spread to lymph nodes. Curable upon early detection.
Melanoma	Begins in the melanocytes in the epidermis. Can metastasize, spreading to even distant cells. Curable if caught before it metastasizes. Difficult to treat after it metastases or spreads.

Melanoma

Superficial melanoma	Most common type of melanoma. It is localized but can travel within the upper stratum corneum layer of the skin before it begins affecting the deeper layers. The first sign is usually flat or only slightly raised with irregular borders and possibly discolored in shades of tan, brown, black, red, blue, or white. Could be found anywhere on the body but most often on the legs of women, trunk of men and on the upper back of both men and women. Most melanoma found in young people is superficial.
Lentigo maligna	Another localized form of melanoma found close to the surface, but usually in the stratum corneum layer of the epidermis. Most often flat or mildly elevated and discolored as tan, brown or dark brown. Usually found in the elderly in skin areas of excessive past sun exposure, including on the face, ears, arms and upper trunk. This is the most common form of melanoma found in Hawaii.
Acral Lentiginous	More invasive form of melanoma found close to the surface in early stages. Usually appears as black or brown under the nails, under the feet or on the palms. Sometimes found in dark-skinned people and is most common in people of African and Asian descent.
Nodular Melanoma	Found in 10-15% of cases and is the most aggressive and invasive form of melanoma. The color is usually black but also can be blue, gray, white, brown, tan, red or skin tone. Malignancy is recognized when it becomes a bump.

It is very wise to seek out a skin care specialist, esthetician, dermatologist, or plastic surgeon who knows the early signs of skin cancer. Progressive skin care specialists have a digital camera they can use to document suspicious growths on your body. Ask your skin care specialist to share those pictures of your skin they use to determine how growths look that might indicate they are cancerous.

The Wellness Approach

After consulting with your doctor, be certain that you cannot reverse the condition and normalize it with a Total Oxidation Management approach before having it removed. Most doctors will give it four weeks before they feel a serious need to remove it. As soon as you witness a growth, no matter the size or the shape, immediately attack it with 12% L-ascorbic acid Vitamin C followed by 5% natural Vitamin E.

I have seen many keratosis affected skin that look and feel as a pencil eraser. They get bigger and bigger in a few days. However, after attacking them with Vitamins C and E for no less than two, and preferably three times a day, I have seen them actually dry up and fall off in four to five weeks.

My personal experience of this was many years ago when a doctor informed me that he had been able to take what he referred to as "pre-cancer" spots off his skin in less than 10 days. He said they just flaked off. We have heard of other cases of people who consider their skin normal weeks after they noticed a growth and began keeping it "In the Mode" with Vitamins E and C.

If it is determined the growth is serious enough to have removed, you now have a "window" for Ultra Violet light to get in and transform healthy cellular molecules into free radicals. Once it's removed, there is no way for the skin to block even short exposure to the sun. "Pull the shades" on that area by keeping that spot "In the Mode;" that is, covered with a layer of freshly-activated L-ascorbic acid Vitamin C followed by a 5% natural Vitamin E solution. If you are going to be outside for a significant amount of time, include a SPF 15 sunscreen for additional protection.

Caution: Total Oxidation Management of Tumors May Surprise You

When tumors begin to develop inside the body, many of the principles of Total Oxidation Management shift. While antioxidants such as Vitamin C are very important in the management of oxidation, once a tumor begins to grow, Vitamin C has been found to help protect the tumor.

This might seem very strange until you remember back in the early chapters when we discussed the findings regarding the most important role of Vitamin C in nature. Vitamin C is found in the highest concentrations around newly developing cells, such as seeds or fetuses. It appears that Vitamin C recognizes a tumor as a newly developing cell and surrounds the cell to protect it and allow it to grow.

This is the reason so many medical professionals warn patients to avoid internal supplements of Vitamin C and excess fruits and vegetables prior to radiation therapy. Just as Vitamin C can protect the skin from sunlight radiation, Vitamin C can protect a tumor from the radiation therapy designed to destroy the tumor.

Lionel's Success

Lionel says he never thought much about the sun; he just enjoyed every activity that had to do with sun and water. He admits to getting his share of sunburns, including a very memorable one around age 18. He's from South Africa and has sailed and water-skied for 20 years. His lone concession to the sun's burning rays was to wear a wide-brimmed water hat.

As he started getting older, Lionel noticed spots on his face and decided it was time to check in with a dermatologist. After shining a bright light on his skin, the doctor suggested a cream to help remove pre-cancerous cells.

After two weeks of using that cream, Lionel decided he wanted to try something else. His job with a skin care distribution company to professional salons gave him an opportunity to attend a seminar with Tom Porter from Malibu Wellness for the EC Mode® Vitamin C and Vitamin E product line.

Lionel met with Tom and asked for advice. Tom's recommendation to Lionel - don't wait for the spots to harden, use Total Oxidation Management now, beginning with the *EC Mode® Vitamin C Serum.*

"I would have to say that there was something like a reversal of the sun damage after using the *EC Mode® Vitamin C Serum* and *EC Mode® Hydro-Driver Moisturizer* after I started using it," Lionel says. "My face is much better and even seems to look and feel softer. With the ointment that I got from the doctor, my skin actually broke out, and I've seen that result on my friends of mine from the yacht club who also have the same sun damage. The spots sort of hardened on their faces after blistering before they finally fell off."

"With the Vitamin C on my skin, the spots just healed and went away. I've been using the *EC Mode® Wrinkle-Less Kit* with the *EC Mode® Vitamin C Serum* for about four or five months." He also uses the *EC Mode® Silk Sunscreen* to help offer more protection.

"It's interesting because I'm not the only one to notice. People who know me have commented that my skin looks so much better. Every single one of my customers has commented about the difference in my skin. I'm now trying some of the *EC Mode® Optimum Hair Growth* products on my scalp.

"So instead of just selling this as just another product line, I've become a regular customer myself, and I've been in the salon product business for a while. I keep buying the kits for myself when I run out, so I use the *EC Mode® Vitamin C Serum*, the *EC Mode® Hydro-Driver Moisturizer* and the *EC Mode® Essential Eye Toner* in the *EC Mode® Wrinkle-Less Kit.* Maybe I wouldn't have run across this line if I hadn't already been in the industry, but I'll tell you very honestly, now that I know it's available, I'll always use it. People tell me that they think I'm in my mid-fifties and I'm 68 years old!" he laughs.

Sunburn

Sunburn is a major focus of Chapter 10. The effect sun has on the skin is the most dangerous environmental issue which determines how fast we show signs of aging.

Simply, the UV-B rays that are considered the radiation that causes sunburn to the layers of skin have the ability to zap electrons from healthy molecules in skin cells. When this spark of oxidation occurs and the free radicals are formed, sunburn is the result. The inflammation, tenderness, and eventual peeling of the skin are the result that aggressive and even subtle exposure by the sun can have on skin in a very short period of time.

The Wellness Approach

The most important aspect of Total Oxidation Management is to prevent the exposure of sun that can cause free radicals caused by UV-B rays. Your skin should always be covered with stable Vitamin C and Vitamin E. Additionally, if you are going to have any extended exposure, even up to thirty minutes at a time, the use of a broad-spectrum sunscreen should be applied right on top of the vitamins. Sunscreens should be used only during the day and caution should be taken on how much is used. Most often, a product with a SPF 15 is very sufficient to provide protection available from FDA approved sunscreen ingredients. Many people have reactions to the high concentrations of some of the ingredients; therefore, be smart in your choices and always use in conjunction with the topical application of vitamins.

If you experience sunburn, hope is not lost. It was once thought that once your skin was sunburned, there was no immediate repair. Now we know that the free radicals continue to form and spread from over-exposure to the sun. Therefore, if the skin becomes inflamed, immediate use of Vitamin C in a 12% concentration followed by 5% natural Vitamin E can provide relief by "donating" an electron to the spreading of free radicals, reducing the effects the sun might have on the skin. The 2 steps, in 2 minutes, 2 times a day will provide relief to the feel and appearance of the sunburn. This is also very safe for children and possibly even more important, since most signs of aging are a result of oxidation that occurs when we are young.

George's Success

"As a man, you don't get that much exposure to skin care products while you're growing up," laughed George of Dallas. However, his job caused him to break with American tradition and become an expert in the field of skin and hair care. After he became a top executive for a national department store's salon division, George made it a priority to learn as much as he could about the science of products that are sold in department stores and salons.

That's how he became aware of Total Oxidation Management from Malibu Wellness, one of the salon suppliers. George stated, "What fascinated me about this company's unique concept was the depth of new science and unique education. Out of all the ingredients and products being "sold" to me by our suppliers, no one but Tom was talking about managing the oxidation and free radicals on skin with Vitamin C and Vitamin E. As Tom continued to send me more research on Total Oxidation Management using these vitamins, I took it upon myself to begin reading and learning what I could about Vitamin C and Vitamin E. Soon it was clear to me that the information Tom was sharing with me and the professionals in our salons about his unique delivery of Vitamin C and Vitamin E for the hair and skin was real!"

"I am a little unique because I was in the industry," George continues. "Because of the company I represent, I have had access to people at industry conferences and learned about the ozone layer and the sun." Just as George began testing the EC Mode® products, George had the opportunity to prove to himself the value of Total Oxidation Management and Vitamin C in protecting the skin against free radical damage caused by oxidation from the sun...he got sunburned.

"I knew that you need some type of protection 24 hours a day. But without realizing it, I had stayed out in an overcast day in Dallas, Tex. It was over three years ago and I was working in the yard all day. I had my face protected, but my neck and arms got very burned. I remembered what Tom said and decided to put Total Oxidation Management to the test; so, I applied the *EC Mode*® *Vitamin C Serum* on my neck, but I didn't put it anywhere else, " George reports.

"What was interesting was that in about four or five days my arms were peeling and the neck never peeled. I was absolutely amazed. I told Tom I have given his product the test under the worst conditions. You don't have to be too smart to realize something is happening when you apply these products to the skin."

Total Oxidation Management made sense to George. "There's got to be a better way to get results on your skin than to shock it or peel it on a consistent basis, and that's what so many suppliers were advocating." George just kept hearing Tom's opinion that normalizing the skin was so much healthier than alpha hydroxy acids such as glycolic and peels that radically exfoliate the skin.

What frustrated George as he learned more and more about the beauty industry is the expense of ingredients that sound impressive, but not very effective. Unfortunately, he's seen a lot of that in the personal care industry. "Most of these product lines have exotic sounding ingredients, but there is little science behind them. Yet they charge as much as $100 an ounce for one bottle, without sound scientific data to back up their claims. Show me the scientific data!" George exclaims.

George has discovered that personal care is a lifestyle issue. "There's a lot of clutter in the skin industry... a lot of extra products that you really don't need. Not only does it drive up the cost, but also, busy people don't have time to go through five or six steps a day. Besides, a person needs to use good skin care products their entire life and it has to be viable and affordable for everyone. Less than five percent of the population can afford an expensive product everyday; so it isn't really a viable product. That just doesn't make sense."

The other aspect of the EC Mode® product line that George appreciates is the fact that the Total Oxidation Management team has continued to refine and improve the product line and its delivery system over the years. Total Oxidation Management expands as new skin research becomes available.

George had the opportunity to test a newer version of the *EC Mode® Vitamin C Serum*. Once again, he had spent too much time in his own yard not realizing areas of his skin needed protection. "Saturday night we had a hail storm, and Sunday I got up and went out at 9 a.m. and I shredded trees outside most of the day. Guess what... I burned my neck again. I had not applied the 12% *EC Mode® Vitamin C Serum* to the back of my neck; but when I realized I was sunburned, I immediately applied the Vitamin C and the sunburn was so much better right away, and there was no peeling days later. The way that I look at it, if this stuff works that well after exposure like that, imagine how good it is for my skin every day."

"I think everybody should use these products. And they are especially important for men who are exposed to the elements. We were never taught that we should take care of our skin. I think this product is terrific and I see how they have worked on me for the last three years. I use them every day as my skin care and when I need to repair unprotected skin that was overexposed. I love that I only need the two core products that use the fresh-dried Vitamin C and natural Vitamin E. In all my research, I never saw products do for skin what EC Mode® has done for me."

Swimmers' Oxidation

Swimmers are some of the most flexible and toned people, yet upon inspection of their skin, there are signs of aging that includes lines, wrinkles, and many forms of keratosis and comedones.

Swimmers are likely the most oxidized group of exercise enthusiasts because of their exposure to oxidizers such as chlorine or bromine in conjunction with the calcium, copper, and other minerals in the water where they swim.

During the summer, many swimmers compound their oxidation in outdoor pools that accelerate the damage to their skin. Then to add to the problems for swimmers, the constant wet/dry cycle speeds up the oxidation of skin. Also, swimmers often complain that their skin is dry and itching. That is a reaction from the oxidizing chemicals and minerals on the skin. Total Oxidation Management can change lives for swimmers and those who soak in hot tubs.

The Wellness Approach

It is advised to get "In the Mode" before you enter the pool to minimize the first exposure to harsh elements in the pool. Try to avoid allowing your skin to dry with the pool water still on your skin.

Applying the freshly-activated stable L-ascorbic form of Vitamin C followed by 5% natural Vitamin E will immediately stop the oxidation of the chemicals that would otherwise remain on the skin allowing oxidizing free radicals to form on. We recommend hair products for swimmers' hair and scalp that also include fresh-dried vitamins, as well as shampoos and conditioners for daily use. However, it is important to remember that swimmers seldom have dirty hair or skin. And certainly, exfoliation services would be a huge mistake for swimmers as a lifestyle option due to their over-exposure to oxidation and free radicals.

Find out if chlorine or bromine are used in your pool or spa, and ask that the hardness level be tested in the pool to determine the amount of calcium you are exposed to.

Lucy's Success

Lucy just attended her 30th college reunion in Nashville, Tenn. and she thoroughly enjoyed herself. "I looked around the party at my college friends who graduated around the same time as I did, and I felt really good about myself. " She had been the Homecoming Queen and when she realized she was the only woman who was not wearing make-up, she confirmed to herself the reasons she continues to use the EC Mode® skin care regimen for the past four years.

In college, Lucy discovered swimming as her choice exercise. "I have been swimming off and on for over 30 years. I have always enjoyed being outdoors. I have always been a runner and played tennis, but some of my best physical and mental exercise comes when I swim."

Lucy and her husband decided to build a pool in the side yard and soon their son and daughter became very strong competitive swimmers featured in national swimming magazines. They became the classic "swim family" that commits early mornings, late afternoon, and every weekend to the sport. "We have met some of the greatest people in our life through swimming events, and all of our family still love to swim."

Lucy has been very familiar with the oxidizing chemicals used in her pool, and over time, she realized that there might be a price to pay for swimming so much in such an oxidizing environment.

"When I turned 40, I was seeing the color of my skin begin to change, lines were forming and I was feeling self conscious. I was trying different skin care products depending on what I read or heard most recently that seemed logical and potentially right for my skin," says Lucy. "Fortunately, we were all using sunscreen, but sunscreen is difficult to keep on your skin all the time with all the activity around the pool." Over the next 10 years, Lucy looked in the mirror and saw herself continue to age.

Around the time Lucy was turning 50, she was in a discussion about skin care with a friend she knows and respects in her community. Her friend told her that Malibu Wellness pioneered a new technology in skin care and she thought it would be perfect for her skin. "My friend was using Malibu Wellness products and she was over 70; her skin looked great. And since my family had been using the *Malibu 2000 Swimmers' Action* hair care products for years, I trusted the products." On her next order of Malibu 2000 hair care products, she ordered *EC Mode® Vitamin C Serum* and *EC Mode® Hydro-Driver Moisturizer*. That was four years ago and she has been using them every day since.

"The fact that I do not wear make-up should tell you how I feel about these products. And my daughter uses these same products every day." Her daughter understands Total Oxidation Management and how swimming pool water as well as the sun and other elements in the environment can damage the skin. "Starting as young as she has, I am confident my daughter will age even slower than I did. I am feeling really good about my skin and am looking forward to the next reunion," laughs Lucy.

Wounds

Whether caused by a sudden trauma, such as a cut from an accident or surgery, or by chemical services to treat over-oxidized skin conditions, a wound can be something that heals completely or becomes a permanent new "sign" of trauma on your body.

Depending on the severity of a wound, the healing process may take days, weeks, or even months. The stages of wound healing include:

- **Inflammatory Phase** - This first phase of wound healing is approximately two to five days and consists of inflammation on and around the wound area.

- **Proliferative Phase** - This phase of wound healing last approximately two days to three weeks. Fibroblasts lay bed of collagen (connective tissue of skin) and the wound edges pull together to decrease the wound and epithelialization occurs.

- **Remodeling Phase** – This final phase of wound healing can last three weeks to two years. New collagen forms which increases the strength to the wound area and scar tissue may form. The more severe the wound the more likely a scar may form.

The Wellness Approach

Flying into the windshield at 65 miles an hour is a good place to test the benefits of Total Oxidation Management of wounds—over 45 stitches worth. As I learned in my own experience, a wellness approach includes both a defensive and offensive approach.

It is most important to realize that any wound has the potential for infection. Therefore, care should be taken to defend the wound against bacteria or viral infections that could enter the wound early in the healing process. Therefore, follow your physician's recommendations regarding infection.

Defense also includes protecting the wound against free radicals that might enter the skin during the healing. A wound usually involves the exposure of skin layers below the protective stratum corneum. Therefore, care should be taken to cover those areas from any aggressive oxidation and sunlight exposure.

For an offensive play to help the skin renew, and to improve the appearance of the wound healing, we suggest the freshly activated L-ascorbic form of Vitamin C followed by a 5% concentration of natural Vitamin E to help in all stages of wound healing for the following reasons:

- Due to their anti-inflammatory properties, Vitamin C and Vitamin E can help reduce inflammation in the early stages of wound healing

- Vitamin C can help skin regenerate by increasing collagen synthesis (the connective tissue of skin)

- Vitamin E can improve the healing process of the wound

- Vitamin E can help inhibit scar tissue formation

Jami's "Scar" Success

Jami lives in sunny Tuscon, Ariz. and loves to be active. She believes in exercise and team sports. Unfortunately, two of her sports left Jami with injuries to her knee; a torn meniscus from playing soccer and a torn ACL ligament playing football.

In 2001, she underwent arthroscopy, which left her with three incisions on her left knee. "The incisions themselves were actually painful. It didn't seem like they were healing properly or at least fast enough for me. A week after the procedure, I still had stitches and the next morning I got up and my stitches actually opened up. The doctor told me to keep putting Neosporin on it and just keep it clean. But they hurt so much on their own; it was definitely sore."

All in all, 2001 was not a great year health-wise for the athletic Jami. "This was actually my 16th surgery for the year."

She knew what to expect in terms of scarring from the doctors and from her own experience. "Usually when you have an incision that wide open, it would be dark purple and even protruding and leave a raised scar, and I didn't want that!"

As it turns out, Jami's job ended up helping her prevent that scarring from happening to some of these incisions from the surgeries. Jami is a Sales Representative of skin and hair care products to professional salons in Arizona. When her company decided to represent the product lines of Malibu Wellness, Jami was given an opportunity to attend a Total Oxidation Management seminar given by Tom Porter.

"When he gave the seminar, I remember Tom Porter actually saying that the fresh dried Vitamins C and E would help heal and prevent scarring. I was pretty interested. I understand that the Vitamin C could cause slight sensitivity to the wound initially but that it would subside after daily repeated application. I decided at that point that I should try it. I asked my doctor about it and he said that Vitamin C is good, but, it depended upon the quality of the product."

Jami decided to try her own experiment to test on her own skin the difference the *EC Mode® Vitamin C Serum* could make. "I started with only applying the *EC Mode® Vitamin C Serum* on one particular incision, which was actually the worst one. I applied it three times a day; once in the morning, once in the afternoon and once in the evening, with the *EC Mode® Hydro-Driver Moisturizer* applied to the wound right afterward," she says.

"To my surprise it really didn't burn or sting at all! Since I really wanted to see the difference for myself, I decided to just apply the *EC Mode® Vitamin C Serum* on one incision, and leave two incisions alone without applying it."

The rapid results caught her off guard. "I was very surprised. I actually had a visit with my doctor after I had tried this experiment and he was also very surprised! I had kept applying the *EC Mode® Vitamin C Serum* for about 4 days to that one incision, and it just healed up in four days!"

Jami had decided she had seen enough to convince her she wanted the other incisions included in her Total Oxidation Management plan. "I started using it on the other incisions about four days later and they also healed in two days. The worst one that should be very noticeable now only has a very small scar, more like just a little incision."

"I know it made a difference because I know how fast it healed and it hadn't healed at all in that first week before."

Jami decided to document her experience, but unfortunately, doesn't have a picture from day one after the surgery. "I didn't take a before picture immediately, but I took one the fourth day of when I started using the *EC Mode® Vitamin C Serum* on both sides. And you can see that even my worst incision isn't bad now."

"It's helped, it really has!" So much so, that she's started using the same *EC Mode® Vitamin C Serum* on her face to manage other oxidation problems. "I use the *EC Mode® Vitamin C Serum, EC Mode® Hydro-Driver Moisturizer* and *EC Mode® Facial Cleanser* twice a day on my face. I've used the kit (*EC Mode® Wrinkle-Less Kit*) long enough now to notice that my sun damage is fading."

She's now busy educating her clients, family and friends about the importance of Total Oxidation Management, especially after her own experience with the wounds on her knee convinced her after just four days of use. "When we first got distributorship, I started spreading the word. Even my husband uses the EC Mode® skin care line!"

"These EC Mode® products really do work, and my own extended family members have noticed. My stepmother is a Mary Kay® distributor, and my own mother has been a long-time fan of Lancôme®, but they both acknowledge that EC Mode® is a pretty cool line!"

Wrinkles, Fine Lines & Signs of Aging

This book is mostly dedicated to the conditions around us and within our skin that causes us to show signs of aging. Similar to a tree that has a ring for each year of growth, we have other signs that indicate how long we have been here on this earth.

Your exposure to the UV-A and UV-B rays of the sun throughout your life will cause damage to the outer layer of your skin, resulting:

- extra lines and wrinkles
- age spots, or as I prefer to call them, oxidation spots.

These are the conditions that can make your skin look years older than your age, and both are primarily caused by one source – oxidation by the sun.

The outer layer of skin is profoundly influenced by sunburns and suntans, but the damage goes deeper as the skin tries to protect itself by producing more melanin or pigment, which results in something we call an "age spot."

Age Spots

The first age spot you'll likely notice will be on your hands, because that's an area that gets repeated exposure to the sun. Age spots (sometimes called "liver spots") can also appear on your face, feet, back, and chest – anywhere that gets repeated oxidation damage from the sun.

If you need further proof of what repeated oxidation does to your skin, just compare the top of your hand to the skin on your bottom, or even the skin on the underside of your arm. "First hand" proof that exposure to the sun - or oxidation - is leading to free radical damage, right before your very eyes.

Wrinkles

Meanwhile, the "cushioning" effect of collagen, the substance that literally supports your skin, is also attacked by the damage of oxidation. When collagen is undermined by free radical damage from the sun's penetration of your deeper cellular level, your skin will show it by sagging and the development of wrinkles or fine lines from UVA rays. In other words, wrinkles don't have to be part of your aging process, if you protect your skin from the radiation of UVA rays and the oxidation of your skin.

Obviously, the best defense against wrinkling is prevention. However, if your skin has already been oxidized or aged by too much exposure to the sun, it is good to know that using nature's own defense system can actually repair some of the damage.

Fresh, active, Vitamin C can perform as a "Free Radical Fixer" and help stabilize your skin's condition to prevent further problems as well as stimulate and promote the growth of new collagen to help your skin look younger as it "plumps" out areas that show signs of sagging.

The Wellness Approach

- Scavenge oxidizing free radicals from the sun's ultraviolet rays that darken skin pigment causing age spots.
- Normalize exfoliation of skin to improve skin clarity.
- Provide a barrier to prevent the formation of free radicals.
- Gently acidify the natural pH balance of the skin.
- Increase collagen synthesis for new cell growth.

When we understand the sun actually takes away our own skin's storage of anti-oxidants, doesn't it make sense to put them back on the skin?

Absolutely! That's why so many products have jumped on the anti-oxidant bandwagon. But as we've pointed out previously – just because the label says it has vitamins C and E does not mean the formula inside is:

- Strong enough - You need at least a 10% solution Vitamin C and 5% of Vitamin E to perform maximum benefits
- Fresh enough – Unfortunately, vitamin strength can deteriorate rather quickly unless proper precautions are taken. For maximum potency, mix fresh-dried Vitamin C crystals at home just before use. After mixing, Vitamin C should be kept out of direct sunlight and can even be refrigerated to prolong shelf life.
- Stable and in a good delivery system for the skin – topical Vitamin C is not effective at all unless the pH level is correct (around a 3 in order to normalize the exfoliation of the skin). Currently, many of the Vitamin C products on the market have a high acid pH, which means that the benefits you receive are more for the prevention of free radical damage. But topical Vitamin C has much more to offer.

If you're spending your hard-earned money for your Vitamin C serum – you should demand MORE benefits! Because when all of the pieces of the puzzle are properly put together, you can get actual PERFORMANCE BENEFITS from applying Vitamin C to your skin and hair.

The Benefits of Fresh, Active Vitamin C in an Effective Formula:

1. Diminishes fine lines and wrinkles.
2. Fades age spots that are caused by free radicals during oxidation.
3. Supports optimal conditions for healthy hair and scalp.
4. Increases the synthesis of collagen.
5. Helps speed the healing process

It's obvious that you need to carefully examine the label of the product you're buying and notice the details regarding the formulation (does the label tell you the strength of the vitamins?), the freshness (is it something you mix at home, or does it have a freshness date?), and the delivery system.

Donna's Success

Like most of us, Donna had a couple of skin conditions that bothered her. In trying to address one issue with a product targeted to "fix" the problem, it would be pretty easy to aggravate another.

For example, Donna started seeing small lines that she attributed to cigarettes and sun exposure. "I smoked for about 15 years and I did have some of those smoker's lines – not that many – but still, I could see some," she says.

Her other skin issue was one that looked liked a sunburn – but wasn't. The extra pinkness or blushing in her face was followed by little bumps that looked like acne. She made an appointment with a doctor in the autumn of last year. "I was developing blotches that looked like pimples but were not pimples and so I went to the dermatologist and was diagnosed with rosacea. I was given a prescription called Metrocream and antibiotics. I used the cream two times a day and nothing really happened. It diminished a little bit but didn't go away."

"I started using the *EC Mode® Wrinkle-Less Kit* and saw results in 2 days. It was amazing. My skin felt smoother, looked healthier and I didn't need to use any of the creams I was prescribed. In fact, I have not used any of the prescription any more. People aren't looking at me like I have sunburn anymore. I can't say enough about the product because it has changed my outlook. It really normalized my skin."

She was pleased to find that the *EC Mode® Wrinkle-Less Kit*, which includes the *EC Mode® Vitamin C Serum, EC Mode® Vitamin E Hydrodriver Moisturizer,* and *EC Mode® Essential Eye Toner,* addressed all of her problems – fine lines, sun damage, and rosacea.

"I'm only 33 but I really think that has really helped my skin look younger. It has helped smooth out my wrinkles. I think it helped me stay the age instead of looking older than I am. I also used it on my chest because I had some scarring from sun damage and some incredible results from that too."

It's impressive to her that a high quality, fresh *EC Mode*® *Vitamin C Serum* could address so many problems and still be affordable. She knows the difference between an active, fresh Vitamin C serum and one that isn't stable and has already turned yellow from oxidation. She's a firm believer in *EC Mode*®'s *Wrinkle-Less Kit*.

"I love the product. I love any time I can talk about it. I went to a cosmetic counter and I saw a bunch a C serums on the shelf and they were already discolored. I could tell that they were not active and they were $125 dollars. I couldn't believe it! The proof is in the pudding – the value is there."

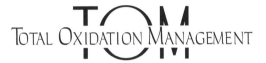

TOTAL OXIDATION MANAGEMENT

In Closing

As you've read, a Total Oxidation Management lifestyle can help normalize many conditions of the skin. Whenever we're asked if this wellness approach can help a particular condition, we always answer, "Give it a try, since we have no indication it can have any negative effects."

We encourage every person with an abnormal skin condition to consult a health care professional if there's an indication of a more significant problem or if they think they have a life threatening condition. However, we always encourage you to apply the vitamins that have been discussed in this book to your skin.

I am confident about the external use of Vitamin C and Vitamin E, and incorporating these vitamins into a lifestyle of Total Oxidation Management. As an educator, it is my responsibility to take new information that is logical and meets the highest standards, and then communicate it to others. If you or someone you know has information that can further develop, confirm, or contradict what is included in this book, please contact me. New information will be used to continue to strengthen our Total Oxidation Management philosophy, and this knowledge will be passed on to others who wish to embrace a lifestyle of wellness.

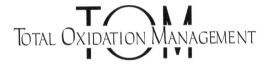

TOTAL OXIDATION MANAGEMENT

Acknowledgments

Lisa Belbot; Teresa Brown; Andres Costo; Patty D'Arrigo; Laurie DeSanto; Paul Dykstra; Kris Gebhardt (author, OVER-HAUL Reinvent, Rebuild and Remake Yourself, GCI Press 2004); Carol Hester; Phil Hester; Marcelo Hochman, M.D. FACS; Jerri Jones; Trish Jones; Nancy King; Mark Krenn; Mary Krupczyk; Dr. Steve Lund; John McCullough; Malibu Wellness Staff; Peggy Porter; Judy Reed; Dr. Rene Reed; Mary Thomas; Charlotte Young, and Dilip Vyas.

References

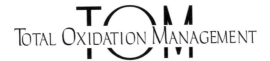

TOTAL OXIDATION MANAGEMENT

References

Chapter 2

Discovery Health :: aging changes in skin. (n.d) Retrieved November 6, 2003 from http://health.discovery.com/diseasesandcond/encyclopedia/497.html

"Creating the Opposite Effect, Scientists Say Anti-Wrinkle Creams May Accelerate Aging," by Lucrezia Cuen, ABC News.com, London, August, 2002.

Why do people have different colours of skin? (n.d.) Retrieved on Monday, November 10, 2003 from http://www.newsandevents.utoronto.ca/bios/askus26.htm

Chapter 3

Interview With Dr. Lester Packer. (n.d). Oxygen Radicals, Pro-oxidants and Antioxidant Nutrients. Retrieved November 6, 2003 from http://www.healthy.net/asp/templates/interview.asp?PageType=Interview&ID=190

Miyachi Y. (1995) Photoaging from an oxidative standpoint. J Dermatol Sci 1995 Mar;9(2):79-86. Department of Dermatology, Gunma University School of Medicine, Japan.

Chapter 4

Denham Harman, M.D. - "Father of the Free Radical Theory of Aging Looks Ahead," by Franklin Cameron. (2003). Retrieved November 6, 2003 from http://www.healthwell.com/hnbreakthroughs/sep98/harman.cfm

Emerit I (1992) Free radicals and aging of the skin. EXS 1992;62:328-41, Free Radical Research Group, University of Paris VI, France.

EXS 1992;62:328-41, Free radicals and aging of the skin. Emerit I, Free Radical Research Group, University of Paris VI, France.

Chapter 5

Dr. Edward D. Harris. (Tuesday October 2, 2001). Oxidants and Antioxidants. Retrieved November 6, 2003 from http://www.geocities.com/bich107g1/

Vitamin A (Retinol) (2002). Retrieved November 7, 2003 from http://www.healthandage.com/html/res/com/ConsSupplements/VitaminARetinolcs.html

Do vitamins in pills differ from those in food? (n.d) Retrieved on Monday, November 10, 2003 from http://www.sciam.com/askexpert_question.cfm?articleID=000DE2DA-7556-1C71-9EB7809EC588F2D7

Zhang L, Lerner S, Rustrum WV, Hofmann GA (1999). Electroporation-mediated topical delivery of vitamin C for cosmetic applications. Bioelectrochem Bioenerg 1999 May;48(2):453-61. Genetronics Inc., San Diego, CA 92121, USA. lzhang@genetronics.com

Niki E (1987). Interaction of ascorbate and alpha-tocopherol. Ann N Y Acad Sci 1987;498:186-99.

Phillips CL, Combs SB, Pinnell SR. (1994). Effects of ascorbic acid on proliferation and collagen synthesis in relation to the donor age of human dermal fibroblasts. J Invest Dermatol 1994 Aug;103(2):228-32, Duke University Medical Center, Department of Medicine, Durham, NC 27710.

Gessin JC, Brown LJ, Gordon JS, Berg RA. (1993). Regulation of collagen synthesis in human dermal fibroblasts in contracted collagen gels by ascorbic acid, growth factors, and inhibitors of lipid peroxidation. Exp

Cell Res 1993 Jun;206(2):283-90. Department of Biochemistry, University of Medicine & Dentistry of New Jersey, Robert Wood Johnson Medical School, Piscataway 08854.

Chung JH, Youn SH, Kwon OS, Cho KH, Youn JI, Eun HC. (1997). Regulations of collagen synthesis by ascorbic acid, transforming growth factor-beta and interferon-gamma in human dermal fibroblasts cultured in three-dimensional collagen gel are photoaging- and aging-independent. J Dermatol Sci 1997 Sep;15(3):188-200. Department of Dermatology, Seoul National University College of Medicine, South Korea.

Davidson JM, LuValle PA, Zoia O, Quaglino D Jr, Giro M. (1997). Ascorbate differentially regulates elastin and collagen biosynthesis in vascular smooth muscle cells and skin fibroblasts by pretranslational mechanisms. J Biol Chem 1997 Jan 3;272(1):345-52. Department of Pathology, Vanderbilt University School of Medicine, Nashville, Tennessee 37232-2561, USA.

Repair, H. Paul Ehrlich, PhD., Harold Tarver, PhD., K. Hunt, M.D. (1972). Inhibitory Effects of Vitamin E on Collagen Synthesis and Wound. Annals of Surgery, Vol.175, No.2, February 1972. Department of Surgery and Department of Biochemistry and Biophysics, University of California, San Francisco.

Traber MG, Rallis M, Podda M, Weber C, Maibach HI, Packer L. (1998). Penetration and distribution of alpha-tocopherol, alpha- or gamma-tocotrienols applied individually onto murine skin. Lipids 1998 Jan;33(1): 87-9. Department of Molecular and Cell Biology, University of California, Berkeley 94720-3200, USA.

Kamimura Mitsuo, Matsuzawa Tohru. (1968). Percutaneous Absorption of a-Tocopheryl Acetate. The Journal of Vitaminology, 1968 June;14(2). Department of Dermatology, Sapporo Medical College for Roche Vitamins, Inc.

August, 1986,Vitamin E Acetate Penetration Studies, Specialty Chemicals Group, Roche Vitamins, Inc.

Puglise, P.:Vitamin E - Skin Smoothness Study, conducted for Hoffman-LaRoche Inc. (1982).

Packer L, Landvik S. (1989). Vitamin E: introduction to biochemistry and health benefits. Ann N Y Acad Sci 1989;570:1-6. Department of Physiology-Anatomy, University of California, Berkeley 94720.

Nachbar F, Korting HC. (1995). The role of vitamin E in normal and damaged skin. J Mol Med 1995 Jan;73(1):7-17. Dermatologische Klinik und Poliklinik, Ludwig-Maximilians-Universitat, Munchen, Germany.

Chapter 6

Paula Kurtzweil (1998). "Alpha Hydroxy Acids for Skin Care: Smooth Sailing or Rough Seas?" *US Food and Drug Administration, FDA Consumer Magazine.* March-April 1998, (Revised May 1999).

Beta Hydroxy Acids in Cosmetics (March 7, 2000). U. S. Food and Drug Administration Center for Food Safety and Applied Nutrition Office of Cosmetics and Colors Fact Sheet. Retrieved November 7, 2003 from http: //vm.cfsan.fda.gov/~dms/cos-bha.html

Chapter 7

What the experts say about indoor air. (n.d.) Retrieved November 22, 2003 from http://www.airstudy.com/experts.html

Chapter 8

Water softeners alternative, water improvements, hard water treatment, swimming pool filters, magnetic water conditioners. (n.d). Retrieved November 6, 2003 from http://www.waterimp.co.uk/

Joe Gelt, Jim Henderson, Kenneth Seasholes, Barbara Tellman, Gary Woodard. (n.d.) Water in the Tucson Area: Seeking Sustainability [Electronic Version]. Retreived November 6, 2003 from http://ag.arizona.edu/ AZWATER/publications/sustainability/report_html/chap6_06.html

The Calcium Factor: The scientific secret of health and youth by Robert R. Barefoot & Carl J. Reich, M.D., copyright 2002.

Chapter 9

Nicole Haralampus-Grynaviski, Carla Ransom, Kerry Hanson, John D. Simon. (n.d.). The In Vitro Photochemistry of Urocanic Acid. Retrieved November 7, 2003 from http://www.photobiology.com/photoiupac2000/ grynaviski/urocanic.html

Ramani M.L., Bennett R.G. (1993). High prevelance of skin cancer in World War II serviceman stationed in the Pacific Theater. *Journal of American Academy of Dermatology,* 1993, Vol. 28:733.

The Skin Cancer Foundation. (n.d.) http://www.skincancer.org/

Alisa Zapp Machalek. (1998). "UV Skin Damage in a Different Light." NIGMS, The National Institute of General Medical Sciences, NEWS & EVENTS, 2003.

Dr. Jan de Winter. (n.d.) Cancer Prevention Advice. Retrieved November 7, 2003 from http://www.dew-health.org/html/skin_cancer.html

"Breakthrough in Sun Protection." (2001) Global Cosmetic Industry (GCI), April 2001.

Melanoma & Skin Cancer (n.d.) Retrieved November 7, 2003 from http: //www.mdanderson.org/care_centers/melanoma_skin/

Johns Hopkins Medical Institutions, Department of Biological Chemistry. (2000). Generalities About Skin Epithelia. Retrieved November 7, 2003 from http://www.hopkinsmedicine.org/CoulombeLabPage/generalskin.htm

J Photochem Photobiol B 1992 Jun 30;14(1-2):105-24, Skin photosensitizing agents and the role of reactive oxygen species in photoaging. Dalle Carbonare M, Pathak MA, Department of Dermatology, Harvard Medical School, Massachusetts General Hospital, Boston 02114.

Guercio-Hauer C, Macfarlane DF, Deleo VA. (1994). Photodamage, photoaging and photoprotection of the skin. Am Fam Physician 1994 Aug;50(2):327-32, 334. State University of New York Health Science Center at Brooklyn.

Taylor CR, Stern RS, Leyden JJ, Gilchrest BA. (1990). Photoaging/photodamage and photoprotection. J Am Acad Dermatol 1990 Jan;22(1): 1-15. Department of Dermatology, Beth Israel Hospital, Harvard Medical School, Boston, MA.

Dalle Carbonare M, Pathak MA. (1992). Skin photosensitizing agents and the role of reactive oxygen species in photoaging. J Photochem Photobiol B 1992 Jun 30;14(1-2):105-24. Department of Dermatology, Harvard Medical School, Massachusetts General Hospital, Boston 02114.

The Relationship between Frequency and Wavelength of electromagnetic spectrum. (n.d.) Retrieved November 21, 2003 from http: //imagine.gsfc.nasa.gov/docs/teachers/lessons/roygbiv/roygbiv.html

Chapter 10

Actinic keratosis, solar keratosis, precancer Patient Information. (n.d.) Retrieved November 6, 2003 from http://www.docderm.com/patient_ information/actinic_keratosis.htm

Dr. K. Stefanopoulos, NCSR Demokritos. (January 19, 2001). NSE studies of water diffusion through the lipid bilayer region in stratum cornem. Retrieved November 7, 2003 at http://www.hmi.de/bensc/report2000/pdf-files/bio-03-0115.pdf

"Sunscreen Drug Products For Over-The-Counter Human Use; Final Monograph," DEPARTMENT OF HEALTH AND HUMAN SERVICES Food and Drug Administration, Federal Register: May 21, 1999 (Volume 64, Number 98)] [Rules and Regulations] [Page 27666-27693] From the Federal Register Online via GPO Access [wais.access.gpo.gov]

Palumbo A, d'Ischia M, Misuraca G, Prota G. (1991 Jan 23). Mechanism of inhibition of melanogenesis by hydroquinone. Stazione Zoologica University of Naples, Italy. Retrieved on Monday, November 10, 2003 from http://www.ncbi.nlm.nih.gov/entrez/query.fcgi?cmd=Retrieve&db=PubMed&dopt=Abstract&list_uids=91120828

Dr. Michael Elstein (n.d.) Eternal Health [electronic version]. Retrieved on Monday, November 10, 2003 from http://www.eternalhealth.org/the_ book/index.html

Darr D, Dunston S, Faust H, Pinnell S, North. (1996). Effectiveness of antioxidants (vitamin C and E) with and without sunscreens as topical photoprotectants. Acta Derm Venereol 1996 Jul;76(4):264-8, Carolina Biotechnology Center, Raleigh, N.C., USA.

Jurkiewicz BA, Bissett DL, Buettner GR. (1995). Effect of topically applied tocopherol on ultraviolet radiation-mediated free radical damage in skin. J Invest Dermatol 1995 Apr;104(4):484-8, Radiation Research Laboratory, University of Iowa College of Medicine, Iowa City 52242-1101, USA.

Nakamura T, Pinnell SR, Darr D, Kurimoto I, Itami S, Yoshikawa K, Streilein JW Schepens (1997). Vitamin C abrogates the deleterious effects of UVB radiation on cutaneous immunity by a mechanism that does not depend on TNF-alpha. J Invest Dermatol 1997 Jul;109(1):20-4. Eye Research Institute and Department of Dermatology, Harvard Medical School, Boston, Massachusetts 02114, U.S.A.

Dreher F, Gabard B, Schwindt DA (1998). Topical melatonin in combination with vitamins E and C protects skin from ultraviolet-induced erythema: a human study in vivo. Br J Dermatol 1998 Aug;139(2):332-9. Maibach HI University of California, School of Medicine, Department of Dermatology, Box 0989, Surge 110, San Francisco, CA 94143, USA.

Darr D, Combs S, Dunston S, Manning T, Pinnell S, (1992). Topical vitamin C protects porcine skin from ultraviolet radiation-induced damage. Br J Dermatol 1992 Sep;127(3):247-53. Duke University Medical Center, Division of Dermatology, Durham, NC 27710

McVean M, Liebler DC. (1999). Prevention of DNA photodamage by vitamin E compounds and sunscreens: roles of ultraviolet absorbance and cellular uptake. Mol Carcinog 1999 Mar;24(3):169-76, Department of Pharmacology and Toxicology, College of Pharmacy, University of Arizona, Tucson, USA.

Kerry M. Hanson and John D. Simon (1998) "Epidermal trans-urocanic acid and the UV-A-induced photoaging of the skin." Department of Chemistry and Biochemistry, University of California, San Diego, La Jolla, CA 92093-0341; and ‡ Department of Chemistry, Duke University, Durham, NC 27708. Retrieved November 22, 2003 from http://www.pubmedce ntral.nih.gov/articlerender.fcgi?rendertype=abstract&artid=27936

Lopez-Torres M, Thiele JJ, Shindo Y, Han D, Packer L. (1998). Topical application of alpha-tocopherol modulates the antioxidant network and diminishes ultraviolet-induced oxidative damage in murine skin. Br J Dermatol 1998 Feb;138(2):207-15, Department of Molecular and Cell Biology, University of California, Berkeley 94720-3200, USA.

Ritter EF, Axelrod M, Minn KW, Eades E, Rudner AM, Serafin D, Klitzman B. (1997). Modulation of ultraviolet light-induced epidermal damage: beneficial effects of tocopherol. Plast Reconstr Surg 1997 Sep;100(4):973-80, Division of Plastic, Reconstructive, Maxillofacial and Oral Surgery, Duke University Medical Center, Durham, N.C., USA.

Fuchs J, Kern H. (1998). Modulation of UV-light-induced skin inflammation by D-alpha-tocopherol and L-ascorbic acid: a clinical study using solar simulated radiation. Free Radic Biol Med 1998 Dec;25(9):1006-12, Department of Dermatology, Medical School, J.W. Goethe University, Frankfurt, Germany.

Eberlein-Konig B, Placzek M, Przybilla B. (1998). Protective effect against sunburn of combined systemic ascorbic acid (vitamin C) and d-alpha-tocopherol (vitamin E). J Am Acad Dermatol 1998 Jan;38(1):45-8, Dermatologische Klinik und Poliklinik der Ludwig-Maximilians-Universitat Munchen, Munich, Germany.

References

Record IR, Dreosti IE, Konstantinopoulos M, Buckley RA. (1991). The influence of topical and systemic vitamin E on ultraviolet light-induced skin damage in hairless mice. Nutr Cancer 1991;16(3-4):219-25, Division of Human Nutrition, CSIRO, Adelaide, South Australia.

Trevithick JR, Shum DT, Redae S, Mitton KP, Norley C, Karlik SJ, Groom AC, Schmidt EE. (1993). Reduction of sunburn damage to skin by topical application of vitamin E acetate following exposure to ultraviolet B radiation: effect of delaying application or of reducing concentration of vitamin E acetate applied. Scanning Microsc 1993 Dec;7(4):1269-81. Department of Biochemistry, Faculty of Medicine, University of Western Ontario, London, Canada.

Thiele JJ, Traber MG, Packer (1998). Depletion of human stratum corneum vitamin E: an early and sensitive in vivo marker of UV induced photo-oxidation. J Invest Dermatol 1998 May;110(5):756-61. L, Department of Molecular and Cell Biology, University of California, Berkeley, USA.

Shindo Y, Witt E, Packer L. (1993). Antioxidant defense mechanisms in murine epidermis and dermis and their responses to ultraviolet light. J Invest Dermatol 1993 Mar;100(3):260-5. Department of Molecular and Cell Biology, University of California, Berkeley 94720.

Chapter 11

The skin. (n.d.) Retrieved November 6, 2003 from http://www.geocities.com/hotsprings/9209/skin.html

W.W. Christie. (6/6/2003) CERAMIDES. Retrieved November 6, 2003 from http://www.lipid.co.uk/infores/Lipids/ceramide/

Keratin and collagen. (n.d.) Retrieved November 6, 2003 from http://www-biol.paisley.ac.uk/courses/StFunMac/glossary/collagen.html

Rebecca James Gadberry. Skin, Inc. Magazine. July 2002, p66-70.

Yaar M, Gilchrest BA. (1990). Cellular and molecular mechanisms of cutaneous aging. J Dermatol Surg Oncol 1990 Oct;16(10):915-22. Department of Dermatology, Tufts University, Boston, Massachusetts.

Tanaka H, Okada T, Konishi H, Tsuji T. (1993). The effect of reactive oxygen species on the biosynthesis of collagen and glycosaminoglycans in cultured human dermal fibroblasts. Arch Dermatol Res 1993;285(6):352-5. Biochemical Research Institute, Nippon Menard Cosmetic Co. Ltd., Gifu, Japan.

The Integumantary System. (n.d) Pensacola Junior College, biology lessons. [Electronic Version]. Retrieved November 7, 2003 from http://itech.pjc.cc.fl.us/fduncan/bsc1093/ap1c5ppt.PDF

Chapter 12

Laser Resurfacing for Facial Skin Rejuvenation (n.d.) Retrieved on Monday, November 10, 2003 from http://www.aad.org/pamphlets/laserresurface.html

Los Angeles Times, HEALTH section, Monday, May 26, 2003, pages F1 and F5.

Laser Resurfacing Aging and Scars. (n.d.) Retrieved on Monday, November 10, 2003 from http://www.lasersurgery.com/more_laser_resurfacing_aging_and_scars.html

Michael Lehrer, M.D., Department of Dermatology, University of Pennsylvania Medical Center, Philadelphia, PA. (8/15/2003). Skin smoothing surgery. Medical Encyclopedia. Retrieved on Monday, November 10, 2003 from http://www.nlm.nih.gov/medlineplus/ency/article/002987.htm

H. Sharma, M.D., and C. Clark, M.D. (1998). Contemporary Ayurveda by (Edinburgh: Churchill Livingstone, 1998; ISBN: 0 443 05594 7) ghostwritten by Bernard D. Sherman.

Anthony C. Gatrell and Janette E. Rigby, "Spatial Perspectives in Public Health." In M.F. Goodchild and D.G. Janelle (editors), Spatially Integrated Social Science, © 2003 Oxford University Press. Retrieved on Monday, November 10, 2003 from http://www.csiss.org/best-practices/siss/18/siss_ch18_tables.pdf

Chapter 13

Otolaryngology Head and Neck Surgery, Vol. 114, Number 2, February 1996

Find a Surgeon. (n.d.) Retrieved on November 21, 2003 from http://www.bosshardtandmarzek.com/find_surgeon.htm

Requirements for eligibility to take the examination (n.d) The American Board of Dermatology. Retrieved November 21, 2003 from http://www.abderm.org/residency.html

Title 16, Division 9, California Code of Regulations Bureau of Barbering and Cosmetology (n.d) "950.3. Curriculum for Skin Care Course"

Retrieved November 21, 2003 from http://www.barbercosmo.ca.gov/laws/art7.htm#950.3

Chapter 14

Experimental Use Of Retin-A. (1988). Retrieved on November 7, 2003 from http://www.fda.gov/bbs/topics/ANSWERS/ANS00263.html

Retin-A and Wrinkles. (1988). Retrieved November 7, 2003 from http://www.fda.gov/bbs/topics/NEWS/NEW00163.html

FDA Approves Renova To Assist In Reducing Skin Damage. (1996) FDA TALK PAPER. Retrieved on November 7, 2003 from http://www.fda.gov/bbs/topics/ANSWERS/ANS00703.html

FDA Warning Letter, Johnson & Johnson Consumer Companies, Inc. (Retin-A)

Micro (tretinoin gel) microsphere, 0.1%) (12/3/02). Retrieved on Monday, November 10, 2003 from http://www.pharmcast.com/WarningLetters/Yr2002/December2002/J&J1202.htm

AVAGE® (tazarotene) Cream, 0.1% (n.d) Retrieved on Monday, November 10, 2003 from http://www.fda.gov/cder/foi/label/2002/21184s2lbl.pdf

Microdermabrasion Device Firm Receives Warning Letter (February 19, 2002). Retrieved on Monday, November 10, 2003 from http://vm.cfsan.fda.gov/~dms/cos-derm.html

Alster TS, West TB. (1998). Effect of topical vitamin C on postoperative carbon dioxide laser resurfacing erythema. Dermatol Surg 1998 Mar;24(3):331-4. Washington Institute of Dermatologic Laser Surgery, Washington, DC, USA.

The Latest Options in Non-Ablative Skin Rejuvenation Cast a New Light on Treating Aging Skin (March 24, 2003). http://www.aad.org/PressReleases/Weiss-Non-Ablative%20Skin%20Rejuvenation.html

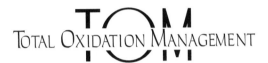

TOTAL OXIDATION MANAGEMENT

Index

Symbols

2 steps in 2 minutes 2 times a day 63, 67, 127, 165
5-alpha reductase 174

A

Ablative Laser Techniques 154
Abnormal skin 58, 133
Acne 62, 65, 149, 150, 173–181
    adolescent 175
    adult 176
    infantile 175
    scars 175
Acral Lentiginous 240
Actic acid 144
Advertising 125
Age spots 20, 44, 45, 58, 141, 146, 158, 182–185
Aging 20, 49, 51, 58, 60, 76, 156
AHA 44, 65, 66, 124, 143, 145, 146, 195
Air 11, 12, 19, 21

Air pollution 46, 70
Air quality 69–74, 72
Alabama 131
Alkaline 82
    ammonias 43
Allergan, Inc. 152
Allergy 140
Alpha-hydroxycaprylic acid 144
Alpha-hydroxyethanoic acid 144
Alpha-linoleic acid 34
Alpha-tocopherol 47
Alpha hydroxy 142, 145
Alzheimer's disease 55
American Academy of Dermatology 148, 211, 222
American Board of Dermatology 130
American Board of Plastic Surgery 130
American Cancer Society 87
American College of Allergists 70
American Dermatology Association 155
American Journal of Dermatology 45
Ammonia 76, 189
Ammonium alpha-hydroxyethanoate 144
Ammonium glycolate 144
Anti-aging 31, 150
Antioxidant 12, 37, 38, 39, 43, 52, 55, 62, 123
Arizona 157, 253
Asparagus 46
Asthma 71
Astringent 64, 65
Athletes 22, 76
Atoms 28, 39
Atopic dermatitis 211
Ault, Keith 4, 39
AVAGE® 152

B

Bacteria 55, 64, 65, 76
Ball State University 4, 39
Basal
    cells 116
    cell carcinoma 239

layer 112, 115
section 111
Bath 75
Baumann, Leslie 148
Becker, David 55
Berkeley University 121
Beta-carotene 108
Beta hydroxybutanoic acid 146
BHA 65, 66, 124, 143, 146
Bicycles 21
Biosynthesis 44
Bleach 22, 29, 71, 76
Blood 46, 55, 81, 105
Blushing 235
Bodily fluids 81
Broken Capillaries 186–188
Bromelain 54
Bromine 248
Build-up 63, 132
Bumps 59
Burning 139, 151
Burns 45, 98, 105
    Chemical 189–192
    Electrical 189
    First degree 140
    Second degree 140
    Thermal 189–192
    Third degree 140
By-products 20, 31

C

C-Free 5, 37
Calcium 54, 77, 78, 211, 248
    hypochlorite 76, 189
California 131
Car 21, 70
Carbon monoxide 72
Cells 35, 41
    oil (fat/lipid) cells 35
    water cells 35
Cell membranes 45

Ceramides 108, 118
Chemexfoliation 141
Chemicals 19, 33, 70
Children 71, 75
Chloride 22
Chlorine 22, 27, 76, 140, 162, 198, 211, 248
Cholesterol 108
Cigarettes 9, 30, 70, 140, 162
    cigarette smoke 27
Citric acid 144
Clay mask 65
Cleansers 63, 64
Cleansing 64
CO2 154
Coal 72
Coarse skin 152
Collagen 13, 49, 50, 63, 107, 125, 139, 156
    remodeling phase 162
    synthesis 43, 44
Comedogenic 62
Comedones 182–185, 248
Complexion 43
Conditions 8
Contact dermatitis 140, 201–204, 222
Cooper, Kenneth 4
Copper 54, 77, 79, 248
Corpuscles 110
Cortisone 67, 205, 217
Cosmetic 132
    beautification 133
Cosmetologists 145
Cradle Cap 198–200
Cuts 105

D

D-alpha-Tocopherol 47
Dandruff 11, 75, 77, 205
Dark Spots 58
Darr, David 40
Day Spa Magazine 160
DA Center for Drug Evaluation and Research 223

Deep wrinkles 152
Delivery system 33, 42
Dermabrasion 156–157
Dermatologist 128, 129, 130, 133, 134, 153
Dermis 44, 63, 90, 91, 107, 109, 140
Desmosomes 116
Detergents 64
DHEA 173
Diaper Rash 208–210
Diet 81
Dihydroxyacetone 101
Dirt 63, 65
Diseases 50
Dissolving 139
Djerassi, David 34, 40
Djhydrotestosterone 173
Dl-alpha –Tocopheryl acetate 47
DNA 28, 29, 91, 239
Doctors 129–138, 136
Dry, irritated hands 71
Dry-cleaning 71
Dryness 151
Dry skin 78
DSM Nutritionals 34
Duke University 40
Dykstra, Paul 131

E

Eczema 11, 75, 77, 78, 205, 211–215
Elastin 44, 107, 109
Elbows 111
Electricity 88
Electromagnetic radiation 88
Electron 20, 28, 38, 44, 49, 53
Elements 19
Environment 8, 10, 67, 69–74, 75–86, 169
Environmental Protection Agency 71
Enzymes 23, 31, 52, 53
    papaya 54
    pineapple 54
Epidermis 37, 41, 58, 90, 109, 140, 141

Erythema 98
Essential oils 52
Estheticians 128, 129–138, 131, 134, 145
Eumelanin 108
European Commission 142
Evans, Herbert 45
Exercise 22
Exfoliation 13, 43, 44, 52, 60, 64, 66, 104, 115, 123–128
   deep 147
   normalizing 127, 165
   radical 124, 126, 127, 139–140, 141, 143, 164
External application 12
Extraction 132, 144
Extracts 33, 52
Extrinsic 9
Eye lift 232

F

Fabrics 70
Facials 131
Fair-skinned 126
Fat-soluble 147
Fats 34, 108
FD&C 132
FDA 34, 51, 132, 145, 244
Feet 111, 119
Fibroblasts 109, 124, 155
Fine lines 44, 58, 141, 255–260
Fine wrinkles 146
Flexibility 22
Florida 131
Florida International University 55
Foods 39, 46
Fossil fuels 72
Fountain of youth 33
Freckles 45, 156
Freeze injuries 190
Free radicals 3, 12, 27–32, 38, 39, 43, 44, 49, 53, 55, 69, 70, 72, 77,
   96, 125, 136, 169
Fruits 106
Fruit acids 33, 52

Fumes 71
Funk, Casimir 34

G

Gadberry, Rebecca 97
Gases 70
Genetics 8
Global Cosmetics Industry 102
Glycolic acid 44, 124, 144, 145
Glycomer 145
Golf 22
Granular layer 117
Grapefruit extracts 52
Grape seed 52
Great Britain 78
Green tea 52

H

Hair 21, 42, 43
    growth 105
    loss 55, 72
Hands 111, 119
    chapped 216
    cracked 216
    Dry 216–221
    Irritated 216–221
Hanson, Kerry 96, 102
Hard water 77, 78, 85
Harman, Denham 7
    Theory of Aging 7
Hayflick, Leonard 164
    Hayflick limit 164
Heart attack 55
Heat 42, 61
Helicobacter pylori 236
Herbs 132
Hiking 126
Home 23
Hormones 58
Horny layer 120
Hot tubs 248

Hydrochloric acid 189
Hydrofluoric acid 189
Hydrogen 22
Hydroxycaprylic acid 144
Hydroxy acids 52, 64
    Alpha 143, 193–197
    Beta 143, 146
Hyper C reaction 45
Hypo-pigmentation 59

I

Impurities 63
INCI 47
Indiana University at Bloomington 3
Indoor air 70
Infant skin 78
Infection 55, 140
Inflammation 30, 43, 65, 98, 135
Infrared-Light therapy 159
International Nomenclature of Cosmetic Ingredients 47
Intrinsic 9
In the Mode 5, 51, 67, 93, 169, 248
Iron 54, 77, 78, 79
Irritation 65, 67, 147
Itching 151

J

Johnson & Johnson Consumer Companies, Inc. 149, 150, 151
Journal of the American Medical Association 150

K

Keratin 107, 118
Keratinocyte 110, 112, 114, 117, 119, 226
Keratin protein 13, 49, 58, 112
Keratosis 59, 136, 182–185, 248
King, Nancy 131
Ko, Hon Sum 223

L

L-alpha hydroxy acid 145

Label 36, 42, 51, 66
Langerhans 115, 117
Larson, Joseph 4, 39
Laser 154
    carbon dioxide 154
    Er:YAG 155
    resurfacing 153
    surgery 186
    YAG 155
Lather 78
Lead 77, 80
Leafy Green Vegetables 46
Lentigo 182
    maligna 240
Light Spots 59
Lime 77, 78
Lines 39, 248
Linoleic acid 34
Lipid 49, 108
    compounds 46
    layers 50
    walls 53
Lipid-soluble 146
Liposomes 40, 42
Liquids 70
Litmus paper 85
Lunch-break peel 157, 193

M

Magnesium 77, 78, 79, 85
Magnets 88
Make-up 63
Malibu 2000 6
Malibu Wellness, Inc 6
Malibu Wellness Institute 53, 143
Malic acid 144
Malonyldialdehyde 49
Marketing hype 33
Master Esthetician 131
Medical devices 132
Medical Procedures 133

Medications 92, 140, 201
Melanin 43, 45, 58, 88, 104, 108
Melanocytes 91, 108, 117
Melanoma 115, 239
Menopause 44
Merkel cells 115
Metabolism 20
Metals 21, 70
Microdermabrasion 124, 157, 197
    home 158
Minerals 33, 52, 54, 77, 85
Mitochondria 31
Mixed fruit acid 144
Moisture 46, 67, 105
Moisturizers 62, 67
Molecule 28, 44, 53, 55, 87
Mud compounds 65
Mud Masks 65
Muscles 11
    stimulation 158
    tone 22
Mutations 28

N

N-Lite® 177
Nail salon professionals 71
Nanosomes 40
Nature 66, 103, 121, 123
Neutrogena Professional division 149
Nitrogen 22, 55
    dioxide 72
Nitrones 55
Nodular Melanoma 240
Non-ablative laser 155
Normalizing 13, 43, 51, 53, 61, 64, 65, 66, 125, 144
Normal skin 57
Nutrition 23
Nuts 46

O

Observation 144

Octyl Methoxycinnamate 98
Oil 62, 104, 108
Olives 46
Omega-3 34
Omega-6 34
Orthotolidine 85
Ortho Pharmaceutical Corp. 149
Outdoor sports 22
Oxidation 1, 2, 12, 20, 21, 39, 58, 69, 73, 168
Oxides of nitrogen 72
Oxidizers 43, 44, 49
Oxygen 19, 20, 69, 76, 167
    free radicals 20
    therapy 159–160
Ozone layer 88

P

PABA 96
Packer, Lester 20, 121
Papillary Layer 110
Pauling, Linus 4
PBN 55
Peels 124, 127, 135, 151
    AHA & BHA 143
    chemical 30, 44, 83, 124, 131, 140, 141–142, 193–197
    medium depth 142
    deep 141
    laser (light energy) 124, 153
    Phenol 147
    radical 161
    superficial 141
    TCA 146
Perms 71
Peroxide 22, 189
PH 33, 42, 43, 44, 45, 64, 65, 66, 72, 80, 81, 85, 102, 143, 145
    acid 41, 43
    Measuring 82
Phaeo-melanin 108
Phenyl Butyl Nitrone 55
Phosphates 189
Phospholipids 118

Phosphoric acid 189
Photo-Aging 43, 44
Photo-damage 150
Photo-sensitivity 140
Photo-toxic 93
Photorejuvenation 156
Pigment 104, 127, 140, 150
    changes 182
    color 45
    disturbances 157
Pinnell, Sheldon 40
Plastic surgeon 128, 129, 130, 133, 134, 153, 232
Poison ivy 201, 222–225
Poison oak 201
Poison sumac 201
Pollution 27, 31, 72, 140, 162
Polycystic Ovary Syndrome 174
Polyglycolic peel 197
Pomegranate 52
Pores 43, 61, 62, 63, 64, 65, 149
Pre-cancer 59
Prednisone 67, 205, 217
Premature aging 37
Printing odors 71
Pritikin Longevity Center 4
Products 60
Professional stylists 71
Protein 44, 54, 125
    cells 104
Psoralen® 227
Psoriasis 11, 75, 77, 205, 226–231
PUVA® 227

Q

Q-10 53

R

Radiation 87, 88
    therapies 29
Radical exfoliant 65
Radical exfoliation 44, 52, 54

Randazza, Lisa 160
Re-epithelization phase 162
Recommended Daily Allowance 34
Reconstructive Surgery 232–234
Redness 45
Rejuvenique® Facial Mask 158
Renova® 151–153
Residue 64
Resurfacing 124, 126
Reticular Layer 110
Retin-A® 150
RETIN-A MICRO® 149
Retinoids 148
Retinol 147
Rhinophyma 235
Roche 47
Room temperature 42
Rosacea 45, 65, 235–238
Rust 21

S

Sagging skin 20, 59
Salicylate 146
Salicylic acid 146, 205
Salon 136
    professionals 71
    service failure 72
Salton 158
Sanding 139
Scalp 21, 42
Scars 20, 50, 140, 146, 157, 253
    tissue 49
Screening 132
Scrubs 66
Sebaceous glands 173
Seborrhoeic Dermatitis 198
Sebum 62, 65, 149, 173
Seeds 46
Self-tanning products 101
Senile Lentigines 182
Shave 67

Shower 75, 81
Signs of aging 20, 156, 255–260
Silicones 61, 62
Simons, John 96
Skin 12, 13, 21, 42, 103–122
    -care professional 128, 129–138, 134
    cancer 28, 87, 88, 96, 116, 239–243
    cells 13
    Components of 104
    growths 239–243
    Inflammation 45
    itchy 72, 75, 77
    layers 39
    redness 151
    texture 36
    The Physical Building Blocks of 106
Smoke 72
Smoking 30, 70, 71
Society of Agricultural Engineers 78
SOD 53
Sodium
    hydroxide 189
    hypochlorite 76
Sodium salicylate 146
Soil 19
Solar
    actinic 59
    comedones 59
Southern California 157
South Florida 158
Spas 136
SPF 97, 98, 126
    15: 98, 151, 244
    30: 98
    45: 98
Spines 116
Spiney layer 116, 117
Spin traps 55, 56
Squamous
    cell carcinomas 59
    epithelium 239
Statue of Liberty 21

Steroids 217
Stinging 151
Straighteners 71
Stratum
    corneum 46, 111, 120
    germinativum 114
    granulosum 111, 117
    lucidum 111, 119, 216
    spinosum 111, 116
Stroke 55
Subcutaneous layer 110
Sugar 42, 143
    fruit 143
    milk 143
    water 43
Sugar cane extract 145
Sulfuric acid 189
Sulfur dioxide 72
Sun 11, 12, 19, 21, 44, 49, 61, 70, 87–94, 140, 142, 162
Sunbathing 92
Sunburn 29, 30, 45, 90, 91, 96, 97, 142, 244–247
Sunlight 59, 72, 152
Sunscreen 49, 50, 95–102, 126, 152
    Chemical 97
    Physical 97
Suntan 90, 91
Superficial melanoma 240
Supplements 23, 34, 39, 46
Sweat 39, 62, 100, 105
Swimmers 22, 76, 126
    Oxidation 248–250
Synthesis 44

T

T-UA 102, 118
Tanning 101
    beds 27, 87, 91
    bulb 92
Tar 205
Tazarotene 152
Tazorac® 152

Tears 106
Tennis 22
Thiele, Jens 121
Titanium dioxide 93
Titanium oxide 97
Toners 64
Tonofilaments 117
Topical application 5, 33
Total Oxidation Management 3, 54, 55, 58, 60, 62, 63, 75, 76, 82,
      115, 127, 135, 136, 160, 168, 170
Traber, Maret 121
Traffic emissions 72
Trans-epidermal 46, 67
Trans-urocanic acid 92
Treatment plant 78
Trethocanic acid 146
Tretinoin 149, 151
Tri-alpha hydroxy fruit acids 144
Trichloroacetic Acid 146
Triple fruit acid 145
Tropic acid 146
Tumors 28, 242

U

U.S. 40
Ubiquinone 53
Ultra-violet light 89
University of California 20, 45, 47, 96
University of Illinois 4, 39, 102
University of Michigan Medical Center 150
University of San Diego 102
University of Wisconsin 40
Urushiol 222
UV-A 90, 95
UV-B 90, 95
UV-C 90
UV rays 27, 45, 87, 89

V

Vegetables 106
Vegetable gum 61

Vegetable Oil 46
Virginia 131
Viruses 76
Vitamins 31, 33–56, 132
    antioxidant 34, 37
    fat soluble 35
    water-soluble 35
Vitamin A 147, 148, 149
Vitamin B 34
Vitamin C 3, 33–56, 61, 62, 64, 67, 101, 106
    12% freshly-activated 5
    active 42
    ascorbyl palmatate 40
    coated encapsulated 40
    freshly activated 41
    L-ascorbic acid form of 3, 31, 33–56, 39, 60–61, 102, 169
    magnesium ascorbyl phosphate 40, 42
    sodium ascorbate 40
    sodium ascorbyl phosphate 40
    stable 41, 42
Vitamin D 34, 88, 105
Vitamin E 3, 33–56, 67, 101
    5% Natural Vitamin E 62
    beta 47
    d-alpha 47
    delta 47
    gamma 47
    Minimum Percentage 48
    natural 3, 31, 33–56, 169
    Natural Form 48
    Stable to Remain Active 48
    synthetic 36
Vitamin F 34

W

Water 11, 12, 19, 21, 70, 73, 75–86, 100
    -element residue 64
    -resistant 100
    -soluble 44, 146
    cells 46, 104
    drinking water 21

Weiss, Jonathan S. 150
Wellness approach 168
Wellness Institute 6
Wet/dry cycle 216, 248
Wheat Germ 46
Willow extract 146
Workplace 23, 71
Wounds 36, 251–254
   Inflammatory Phase 251
   Proliferative Phase 251
   Remodeling Phase 251
Wrinkles 12, 20, 39, 44, 49, 58, 152, 248, 255–260
www.WellnessSalon.com 6, 85

Y

Young, Frank E. 149

Z

Zinc 55
   oxide 93, 97
   pyrithione 205